On The Job With Hearing Loss
Hidden Challenges
Successful Solutions

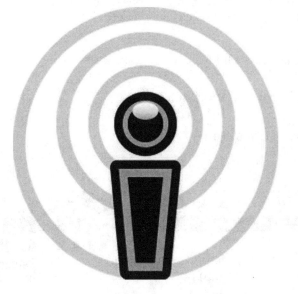

Rebecca A. Morris

On The Job With Hearing Loss

Morris, Rebecca A.
On the Job with Hearing Loss: Hidden Challenges. Successful Solutions / Rebecca A. Morris

ISBN: 978-1-60037-269-8 (Paperback)
Interior Design by:
Bill James, Bill@WAJames.com

Published By:

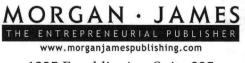

www.morganjamespublishing.com
1225 Franklin Ave Suite 325
Garden City, NY 11530-4943
Toll-Free 800-485-4943

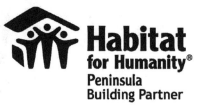

Peninsula
Building Partner

To my heroes, the vocational rehabilitation professionals who change lives every day.

To my family – Bert, Michael and Casey

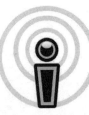

FOREWORD

Industry, professional, and consumer interests have long awaited this insightful and comprehensive resource by my long-time friend and colleague Rebecca Morris. In its pages are hard-to-find yet valuable information about how to meet the challenges of hearing impaired individuals in the workforce. She has gone to great lengths to present examples of just about every listening situation, social circumstance, and managerial challenge possible to show that to ignore this "invisible handicap" is to reap unnecessary loss to the economy (to the tune of more than $112 Billion annually in the U.S. alone!), missed opportunities in promotion and advancement, and additional costs in workplace mishaps.

As one who has struggled for nearly six decades with severe and later profound hearing impairment, I find the author's suggestions right on the mark. As a practicing professional, educator, and researcher in the hearing health field, I find that we have far to go in bringing professionals who serve the hearing impaired up to par in offering the vast array of hearing loss solutions into hearing health practice. Agencies who serve the needs of this same population too often misunderstand the *real* psychosocial and productivity implications, and hence tend to over-promote learned helplessness instead of self-reliance and independence. But, most of all, a vast growing population of hearing impaired consumers--growing in numbers at least as fast as the population is aging--still have to come to grips with the fact that 1) they are missing an important connection to society and to their environment, and 2) there are wonderful and effective solutions to help anyone and everyone to become what I call "communicatively whole".

 How many of the millions who suffer from severe hearing impairment today have yet to go over to their blaring television sets and push that little button labeled "CC"? How many severe-to-profound individuals have yet to discover the communicative empowerment awaiting them with TDD Relay Services on the other end of the telephone line? How many waste their time and money going to amusement parks or neighborhood theatres or concerts because they fail to taking advantage of FM and Infrared listening devices? How many lectures, business meetings, religious services, and musical performances do they attend but aren't really "there", because they don't utilize available, low-cost technologies? If hearing aids and cochlear implants form the foundation, assistive technologies and strategic planning form the walls and roof to communicatively-complete homes, businesses, and public places. Yes, it can be said that hearing loss is one of the most avoidable follies in today's society, if only the available solutions were more taken advantage of by those needing them.

Truly, the hearing impaired population comprises uncountable outstanding, talented, and highly educated individuals who have much to offer society and their employers. As the author so ably points out, even small adjustments and accommodations can make all the difference in the world in productivity, progress, and personal fulfillment.

I encourage everyone--provider, agency, consumer--to make this volume a *primary resource* in the quest to stamp out the folly of hearing loss; to not let it collect dust somewhere on a shelf, but instead for it to be a much referenced guide to *success* in the workplace. Personnel directors need it. Managers need it. Business owners require it. And most of all, anyone experiencing the detrimental effects of lost hearing need their own copy of *On the Job with Hearing Loss* so that they may realize their highest potential in the workplace, in society, and in life itself.

Max Stanley Chartrand, Ph.D.
Managing Director,
DigiCare Hearing Research & Rehabilitation

CONTENTS

Audiologists, hearing instrument specialists, employers, vocational rehabilitation counselors, disability service providers and individuals can all use this book to learn why a systematic evaluation process works to provide effective accommodations for individuals with hearing loss. Discover the special features of this book.

The combination of baby boomers and hearing loss will alter the workforce and the numbers are astonishing. How many people have hearing loss? What is the impact? How do you hire, train and retain a qualified workforce?

How well do you understand hearing loss? There is a hidden cost when dealing with untreated hearing loss for both the employer and the employee. Perceptions, Performance and Pay are all inter-related and can prevent people from reaching their full potential.

Follow a proven method that professionals are using to identify all the issues related to hearing loss and communication. You will be able to perform a comprehensive assessment of all the key areas where difficulties may exist. You can confidently move ahead knowing you have all the data needed to help you find successful solutions. The information that is presented in this chapter is also available as a worksheet that you can copy and use in the back of the book.

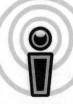

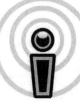

Contents

CHAPTER 9
TECHNICAL SOLUTION #2 - ASSISTIVE LISTENING SYSTEMS
Assistive listening systems provide powerful benefits. You'll understand how these systems work and how flexible they can be to increase their effectiveness. These systems are technical solutions that deserve their own chapter.

CHAPTER 10
We've done the work for you and have lots of information to share. It can't get any easier. You can simply choose an occupation (or one that has similar communication demands) and see the common communication issues and potential accommodations (from non-technical to technical).

Occupations include:

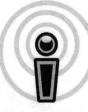

Once you review non-technical solutions and consider hearing aid facts, you will have all the information you need to enable you to secure assistive technology that can help in specific listening situations. Learn about these products that can be "aids for hearing aids".

You may still need guidance in finding the appropriate accommodations for your situation. Since technology changes so rapidly, you'll receive the internet resources that can give you the most current data. The organizations, manufacturer websites and consumer websites will provide the most accurate and up-to-date technical information.

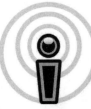

Before You Begin: How This Book Can Help You

This book has been developed from years of experience working with individuals with hearing loss and the professionals who provide services to them. You may be the individual with the hearing loss seeking more information to help you on the job or you may be an employer who must find appropriate accommodations.

If you are a vocational rehabilitation counselor or hearing health professional, you may need technical assistance to help you recommend and choose effective technology.

Are any of the characters in the following story familiar to you?

A Common Story

Jan has been employed for 15 years and has noticed her hearing has changed. She is struggling in many areas that are affecting her job performance. She meets with the company's human resource specialist, Kim. Kim has not worked with an employee with hearing loss and she isn't sure where to start.

Kim goes online and finds an overwhelming amount of data and hundreds of assistive listening and alerting devices. While Kim is gathering data and becoming even more confused, Jan meets with a vocational rehabilitation counselor (Charlie) who may be able to offer guidance and financial assistance with hearing aids.

Charlie sends Jan to the audiologist for a hearing evaluation. Daniel, the audiologist, is able to recommend hearing aids but his practice doesn't include other assistive devices, so he is hesitant to recommend additional solutions.

Everyone has the same goal: find accommodations that will work for Jan. While hearing aids will help in most listening situations, Jan has many communication demands where the hearing aids alone won't provide optimum benefit.

Ideally, any one of these professionals could provide the accommodations Jan needs.

This book would have been invaluable to any one of them. It can help you too.

What Can You Expect?

If you have attended training on assistive listening technology (ALDs), you more than likely learned about the categories and features of the products. You found that the challenge remained 'when and why' to choose a particular product. The learning curve is steep because you need experience to really understand which products are most appropriate.

Tap into years of experience of a professional who has worked with people in virtually every occupation. The goal of this book is to circumvent the learning curve and help you provide the most effective accommodations in the least amount of time.

The primary audience for this book is the employer or professional who has been charged with finding appropriate solutions to help keep an employee productive. However, if you are the person with the hearing loss, you will also gain invaluable resources to help you advocate for accommodations.

If you have limited understanding of hearing loss, you will gain insight into the often invisible barriers to communication faced by people with hearing loss. The chapters are divided so that you can choose the information you need, based on your experience and background.

Who Can Use This Book?

- ◆ Employers and Human Resource Professionals
  - ■ Save time by identifying your resources
  - ■ Learn what you need to know, regardless of your experience
  - ■ Simply choose an occupation and most of the work is already done for you

- ◆ Vocational Rehabilitation Professionals
  - ■ Save time by following a systematic process
  - ■ Compile the same information each time for case documentation
    - ■ Accommodate an employee, regardless of your experience with hearing loss or with technology

- Have the data you need at your fingertips if you seek technology recommendations
- Simply choose an occupation and most of the work is already done for you

◆ Audiologists and Hearing Instrument Specialists

- Understand the typical job functions and environments of an unfamiliar occupation
- Uncover communication issues that may factor into your hearing aid recommendation
- More confidently recommend ALDs that will work with the hearing aid
- Help your patient set realistic expectations of the hearing aids leading to increased success rates and patient satisfaction

◆ Other service professionals who work with individuals with hearing loss and individuals who want to accommodate their own hearing loss

- Learn how to identify all the work issues that may be related to the hearing loss
- Learn basic information on hearing loss and hearing aids
- Become familiar with the technology that may be helpful
- Be better prepared to request accommodations

Why the Process Works

I've spent the second half of my career life specializing in assistive listening and alerting devices, also known as hearing assistance devices. While initially working with vocational rehabilitation counselors to aid in technology solutions for their clients, my services extended directly to the client, the employer and the audiologist because they were all key players with specific information needed for a full evaluation.

As a carry-over from my previous career in systems analysis and technical writing, I developed a process to systematically gather all the data needed from all the parties involved to perform an evaluation. I have used this process with nearly 800 assessments in the past 5 years alone. I know it works.

I want to share with you the systematic process that can help anyone, regardless of their level of experience, lay the groundwork in identifying effective accommodations.

Special Features of the Book

Case studies and examples are included throughout the book to help you understand the human side of hearing loss and technology. Several chapters of the book focus on the most common challenges facing people with hearing loss. An important Resource chapter is included because technology changes at a dizzying pace and you will be able to find the most up-to-date product information and resources.

"Occupations A to Z" is the most unique and innovative chapter of this book. Choose an occupation and learn about the typical job functions and communication issues others have faced. Explore the communication issues and identify those that are similar and learn about common solutions and accommodations.

These reports reflect the experiences of working with hundreds of individuals in every imaginable occupation. I have toured prisons to understand the environments of medium and maximum security facilities, climbed aboard heavy equipment, farm tractors and semi trucks, visited inside hospital operating rooms, factories, warehouses, call centers and every type of work environment imaginable.

This information is action oriented and presents practical steps, tools and resources to identify communication issues on the job.

What This Book Is Not

If you want to learn the differences between hearing aid technologies, you will not find that information within this book. If you want details on the Americans with Disabilities Act or want to learn more about the mental health issues related to hearing loss, you will not find that information here either.

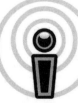

Excellent websites and timely books already exist on these topics. You will find links to this information in Chapter 12, the Resource chapter.

A Final Note

Strategies + Hearing Aids + ALDs = Successful Accommodations

This book is specifically designed to share how communication strategies, hearing aids and hearing assistance products can work together to achieve successful accommodations for people with hearing loss. It is my hope that the information in the following chapters will provide a positive and practical impact on *your* role in finding successful solutions.

Chapter 1 – Hearing Loss is Threatening the Workforce

Beware of a looming threat to the American workforce. Make that a **booming** threat. We've heard the news about the Baby Boomers hitting their prime. The sheer number of boomers is overwhelming and the impact of hearing loss on this generation may be surprising.

The results of a recent Baby Boomer Hearing Loss Survey, conducted in part by the Ear Foundation, indicate that hearing loss is more widespread than previously estimated. This survey states that nearly half of the 76 million baby boomers are experiencing some degree of hearing loss. That's almost 38 million people between the ages of 40-59 who will face the challenges of hearing loss.

The cost of untreated hearing loss is staggering

The Better Hearing Institute estimates that untreated hearing loss costs society 56 billion U.S. dollars each year, mainly due to lost productivity. How did hearing loss catapult to the top of the chart of workplace issues?

One word can describe how many people acquire hearing loss. NOISE. Noise induced hearing loss spares no one. Veterans may have noise induced hearing loss from military service. Baby boomers who enjoyed years of listening to or playing loud music are now noticing hearing loss. The number of people under 40 who will experience hearing loss could be exponential because of the widespread use of earphones for MP3 players and cell phones.

> *Almost 38 million people between the ages of 40-59 will begin to face the challenges of hearing loss*

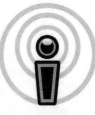

Uncover the hidden costs

Because untreated hearing loss can impact job performance and job retention, people with hearing loss experience higher rates of under-employment and early retirement than the general population. It costs a company significantly more to lose a qualified employee than to accommodate them.

There is also a hidden cost to individuals over their career life-time. Communication challenges can cause mistakes, frustration, misunderstandings, and erode self confidence. This in turn can affect performance reviews, promotions, compensation and ultimately income and retirement contributions.

The tidal wave of an entire generation is gaining momentum and we are preparing to handle the threat. Fortunately the whirlwind of media exposure about baby boomers is creating a positive impact in identifying hearing loss and its impact on quality of life.

So is there any good news?

Yes! Actually, if there is a good time to have a hearing loss, now is probably that time. It is usually true that large numbers of people facing the same problem have a voice. Media attention helps to bring awareness to this issue that will affect you or someone you know.

As far as accommodations are concerned, the good news is that other people with hearing loss have forged the way. A wealth of resources and experiences are available. Professionals who work with people with hearing loss all realize that accommodating a person with hearing loss promotes a win-win situation for both employees and employers.

These resources can have a life-changing affect on someone with hearing loss. Vocational rehabilitation agencies offer professionals who are experienced in assisting people with disabilities. Hearing professionals have an array of sophisticated hearing aid technology at their disposal that can literally transform a person's life. National consumer organizations for people with hearing loss publish valuable information for individuals with hearing loss.

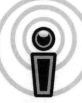

Take the first step

The first step toward successful accommodations is identifying the communication issues on the job. This includes identifying or admitting a hearing loss exists, understanding the potential communication challenges and then investigating potential solutions. You can simply follow the steps laid out by professionals and individuals who have already taken this trip.

Chapter 2 - Profile of Hearing Loss - The Real Impact

Since hearing loss is the number one disability every employer will face, it is important to have a basic understanding of hearing loss and the accommodations that may be needed.

The term hearing loss encompasses anyone with hearing loss and is inclusive of people who are Deaf, late deafened, and hard of hearing with no regard to severity of loss, age at onset, communication methods, use of technology or socio-cultural factors.

We can define three separate groups of people based on their hearing loss and the communications methods that are most effective:

1. **Hard of Hearing**

   This term is used to indicate people who have some degree of hearing loss ranging from mild to profound as defined by audiological measurement. People who are hard of hearing have the following characteristics:

   - Can benefit to some extent from the use of hearing aids or other assistive listening devices.
   - Do not rely on any form of sign language as their primary means of communication.
   - Function in the hearing world with regard to family, friends, work and leisure activities.
   - Do not have significant association with the Deaf community.
   - May or may not have taken steps to deal with their hearing loss (audiological assessment, use of hearing aids or other technology).

2. **Late Deafened**

   This term refers to people who have a severe to profound hearing loss as defined by audiological measurement, which occurred after the development of speech and language. People who are late deafened have the following characteristics:

- Can benefit from the use of visual display technology, but usually derive very little benefit from hearing aids or other listening technology.
- Usually depend upon visual representations of English to communicate with others (may include finger spelling, some system of manually coded English, speech reading, cued speech or written communication).
- May have developed some proficiency in American Sign Language learning as a second language; they function in the hearing world with regard to family, friends, work, and leisure activities.

3. **Culturally Deaf**

   This term refers to individuals who are members of the Deaf community and who use American Sign Language (ASL) as their primary mode of communication. Sign language interpreters are the most requested accommodation.

How well do you understand hearing loss?

True or False: Hearing aids restore hearing like glasses restore sight.

False. Hearing aids amplify all sounds, not just speech sounds. While the newest digital technology can be very helpful to many people in reducing background noise and directional microphones are useful to many depending on their communication needs, hearing aids cannot choose only speech sounds to amplify.

If a person wears hearing aids and is trying to hear someone close to them in a noisy hall, the background noise will interfere in understanding speech. They may be able to hear fine in a small classroom but when the air conditioning fan kicks on, that sound will also be amplified and compete with the speech sound. Our brains learn to filter out background noise, such as the refrigerator running but hearing aids pick up that sound and amplify it, making it difficult to filter out.

True or False: Only older people have hearing loss.

False. Statistics show that in the general population, one in ten people experiences hearing loss. This is across all age groups. The statistics increase in the 40-59 age group to one in two people. The statistics do increase as people age, but hearing loss occurs in people of all ages.

True or False: People with hearing loss are good lip readers.

False. Studies show that even the most proficient speech reader can only pick up about 30% of what is being said. Not all vowel and consonant sounds are visible when spoken.

Speech reading used to be called lip reading. You don't just read lips, you actually read the facial expressions as well. Speech reading helps some people fill in gaps to what they are hearing. The combination of hearing and speech reading helps aid in comprehension.

True or False: When hearing decreases, the other senses evolve to compensate.

False. It may seem that people with hearing loss have enhanced abilities. Their eyesight does not improve. They are actually using visual cues to help them remain aware of what is going on around them and using speech reading to better understand speech.

True or False: Sign language interpreters are the best accommodation for loss.

False. Sign language interpreters are essential to people who rely on American Sign Language to communicate. Most hard of hearing and late-deafened individuals do not know sign language so this is not an effective accommodation for them. Generally, people who are hard of hearing prefer assistive listening systems and people who are late-deafened prefer a visual accommodation such as captioning.

How do you determine if someone has a hearing loss?

Some people hide or try to hide their hearing loss. Others haven't yet accepted their hearing loss. Many just don't know how to improve the communication process. The following behaviors can have a detrimental effect on how a person with hearing loss is perceived:

Bluffing – Pretending to understand, or nodding when they actually don't understand. Many people will bluff because they are uncomfortable asking people to repeat something again and again. It's often easier to bluff than to interrupt and draw attention to their hearing loss.

Distancing – Avoiding social situations and personal contact. Sometimes people will eat lunch alone rather than try to communicate in a noisy lunchroom or with a group of people because it can be hard to keep up with conversations. They may avoid informal social situations for the same reason.

Controlling conversations – Actively work to reduce two way conversations. Some people seem to control a conversation by talking, almost non-stop. This may not even be intentional but it is a way for them to convey what they want to say while reducing the chances of an interactive conversation.

Responding inappropriately – Making a comment out of context to the current topic. In group conversations, they may make a comment that someone else has just made or may ask a question that was already previously addressed. Some people are reluctant to speak up again because of embarrassment and this can increase the likelihood of distancing themselves from certain situations.

The impact of these behaviors can be devastating over time.

The impact of these behaviors can have a cumulative effect on how others perceive the person with hearing loss. Interpersonal relationships may be strained as others may avoid contact with the person with hearing loss. These behaviors are unintentional but the effects can be devastating over time.

Perceptions

Persons with untreated hearing loss may respond inappropriately during a conversation. They may appear unfriendly or 'not with it' to co-workers because they don't answer when someone calls out to them. They may seem anti-social if they avoid informal group conversations.

It can appear they are displaying a lack of initiative or motivation. They may be very hesitant to speak up in meetings to share ideas because of prior embarrassing situations where they may have responded inappropriately. They may make mistakes or hold back from taking a lead role.

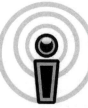

These perceptions may strain personal relationships and cause increased stress on people with hearing loss. They avoid contact which in turn makes them feel isolated. This cycle can erode self confidence and decrease job satisfaction.

Astute managers can often identify employees who may have hearing loss after becoming aware of these hearing loss behaviors.

Performance

Dealing with hearing loss all day can be exhausting, even with all the accommodations possible. It is even more exhausting when individuals are in denial or not yet using hearing aids or assistive devices. In this case, they may not sleep well from waking up every hour to make sure they don't miss the alarm clock. Even worse, they may often be late for work.

Hearing loss is not always considered a significant impairment when, in fact, the person may be suffering from numerous problems and difficulties that are not visibly related to the hearing loss.

Employees may pass up training opportunities or are reluctant to take on new responsibilities because of the communication obstacles they face every day. Sometimes it is hard enough for them to maintain their level of performance, much less take on new responsibilities.

Pay

Persons with hearing loss may receive unsatisfactory performance reviews, based in part from the behaviors they have used to get by. It is a vicious cycle when they try to cope by using ineffective strategies and then their actions are perceived in a negative way.

The cycle may result in poor performance reviews. Poor evaluations affect salary increases. The person with hearing loss may miss opportunities for promotions or supervisory positions. Many people become so frustrated and tired from trying so hard that they give up. Early retirement becomes an attractive option.

> *The most powerful step an individual with hearing loss can take is to learn more about his or her hearing loss and how to successfully live with it. Chapter 12 is devoted to proven resources and methods.*

Why wouldn't a person just get help and buy hearing aids?

Statistics say that it can take a person 7 years from the time they recognize a hearing loss until they actually seek help. There are several factors that may come into play and contribute to this time lag.

People who say, "My hearing loss isn't that bad" are not just being contrary. They may be unaware of the level of loss because when hearing deteriorates over time, they may stop hearing sounds like birds singing and not even recognize the loss. Sometimes they appear to hear every word and at other times they struggle. They have likely been told that it seems they can hear when they want to.

Often it is not the volume or loudness level of speech that causes the hearing difficulty as much as it is the clarity of what people are saying. Some people may be easier to understand than others. Background noise often interferes with the clarity because the person with the hearing loss may only hear parts of words and must try to 'fill-in-the-blanks'. They often miss the first part of a sentence if someone doesn't get their attention first.

Denial is an emotional factor that can delay some people from accepting help. They aren't aware of the level of loss or may fear that wearing hearing aids will be perceived as a sign of weakness or old age.

Hearing aids are an extraordinarily high priced technology. Most people do not have a large amount of disposable cash and the investment seems too great. Other family expenses could have a higher priority, such as buying a car or performing home maintenance. Tuition and other family obligations also come into play.

Stories abound about how hearing aids are not that helpful. It is true that hearing aids don't solve all the problems and may actually aggravate difficulties depending on the listening environment. But hearing aid technology has dramatically improved just within the past 5 years with programmable and digital technology and is worthwhile to try.

What do you mean; "Hearing aids won't fix all hearing problems?"

In general, hearing aids are extremely helpful in almost all listening situations. There are specific times, however, when hearing aids need help to provide optimum benefit. The benefit of hearing aids can be directly related to the communication demands one faces.

A person who does not work or works in a small office may find that hearing aids alone provide significant benefit and no other technology is required. This person does not interact with many people and they are in a good listening environment.

But a person who works in a job with many communication demands, or in what we call an 'unfriendly listening environment', may experience more difficulty and more limited benefit. When interfacing the hearing aid to a telephone or participating in different meetings or trying to hear when background noise is present, hearing aids may be more of a hindrance than a help.

Telephones, meetings and background noise are such troublesome areas that they warrant their own chapters in this book.

OK, so how much will it cost an employer to accommodate an employee with hearing loss?

The cost of accommodations may be much less than most people think. Many solutions involve environmental changes and procedural changes that cost nothing to implement. Simple changes include moving to a quieter workstation to reduce background noise or using meeting rules so that everyone in the meeting can stay on track.

Using products like a phone amplifier or a personal pager can be highly effective in certain situations and are relatively low in cost. Communication access such as sign language interpreters or CART (computer assisted real time captioning) reporters will likely be the highest cost incurred.

Even the highest cost accommodations will reap double dividends to both the employer and employee. The company benefits from increased productivity when providing communication access in a manner that enables a person to communicate, participate and contribute in real time.

Two tax incentives are available to businesses to help cover the cost of making access improvements. The first is a tax credit that can be used for architectural adaptations, equipment requisitions and services such as sign language interpreters. The second is a tax deduction that can be used for architectural or transportation adaptations. See Chapter 12 for more resources on the Americans with Disabilities Act (ADA).

So where do you begin?

There are three general steps an employer can take that will lead to successful solutions:

- Build the team of all the key players.
- Thoroughly identify the communication challenges.
- Seek technical assistance from professionals experienced with hearing loss.

The next steps are laid out plainly for you. Follow them and be led through a proven process that will help you uncover communication challenges, clearly identify where communication breakdowns occur and bring to light the potential solutions. The entire process begins with attitude.

Attitude is defined as a complex mental state involving beliefs, feelings, values and dispositions to act in certain ways. Attitude influences the success (or failure) of implementing changes in the work environment and can be the primary obstacle to successful accommodations. Learn how it can impact the 10 Steps to Successful Accommodations.

Chapter 3 – Ten Steps to Successful Accommodations

Attitude can be the difference between success and failure in all things. This is especially true when dealing with accommodations. As an employer or supervisor, your positive attitude while working towards solutions will impact the work environment for both the employee and his or her co-workers.

All too often, the attitude of co-workers and supervisors becomes a barrier to providing effective accommodations.

The employee's own attitude will also affect the success of accommodations. He or she must feel confident enough to try new technology and become assertive in using accommodations. The work environment and attitudes of others will have a direct impact on successfully using accommodations.

> *A less than supportive work environment impedes the accommodation process and can actually become one of the identified challenges to overcome.*

It goes without saying that a positive attitude can almost guarantee success.

This chapter will lead you in performing a thorough assessment. Each of the following steps has specific directives. Don't skip any of the steps and make sure you answer all the questions. Your answers will uncover the communication demands, determine where the communication breakdowns occur and provide the technical information needed to provide the most appropriate accommodations.

You will use the details gathered here to look for demanding challenges and potential environmental or procedural adjustments. You will be able to provide solutions to many of these issues with adjustments alone.

You will also have the technical data you need when looking for technology solutions.

1. List the essential job functions.

The goal is to look at each job duty and identify all the areas where the hearing loss may be affecting job performance. Often the supervisor will recognize the impact on performance more clearly than the employee (such as inaccurate phone messages with wrong phone number or name).

For example: The critical job duties of a receptionist include greeting clients when they arrive and learning who they wish to see. The receptionist must be able to answer the phone and attend a weekly staff meeting.

The communication demands are 1) Answer the phone and hear on the phone, 2) Know when a client approaches, 3) Hear customers from across the desk or counter and 4) Participate in weekly meetings.

Breakdowns occur when the receptionist cannot hear callers clearly on the phone, cannot hear clients approach when she is on the phone, or cannot hear clients speak across the counter - especially when the copy machine is running in the background. The staff meeting with 15 people is difficult because she cannot hear people at the far end of the table.

a. List the critical job functions or duties

_____

_____

_____

_____

_____

_____

_____

b. List the communication demands of each job function

_____

_____

_____

_____

_____

_____

c. List where breakdowns occur

_____

_____

_____

_____

_____

_____

_____

2. Describe the communication issues when interacting with these groups.

The goal is to identify how well the individual can communicate with each group and list where problems cause undue stress and poor performance. An unidentified hearing loss may be creating problems that are perceived as negative behavioral or interpersonal issues as well as performance issues.

For example:
Supervisor: In one-on-one meetings in the supervisor's office, it is not difficult to hear. When trying to hear when out on the floor, the background noise interferes with understanding.

Co-workers: It is difficult hearing co-workers because they speak low or background noise is present. The individual avoids social chatting or eating with others because it is so difficult to keep up with the conversation. He or she may also report feeling embarrassed because they ask co-workers to repeat often.

Customers: Soft spoken customers are hard to understand. The receptionist may be perceived as rude when she does not answer or acknowledge a customer who walks up behind her. She must ask customers to repeat several times to understand.

a. Supervisor

_____

_____

_____

_____

b. Co-workers

_____

_____

_____

_____

c. Customers

_____

_____

_____

_____

_____

_____

3. Find out information about the hearing aid or cochlear implant.

This technical information is necessary if problems are identified when using the telephone or other device or if background noise is an issue.

For example: The receptionist from Step 1 has relatively new in-the-ear (ITE) hearing aids. The telephone squeals when she places the phone against her ear and the aid does not have a telecoil (or telephone switch). The information needed about the hearing aid is the **model** (Phonak Savia), **style** (in-the-ear), and **options** (telephone switch). Potential solutions will depend on this data.

a. Identify the model, style and age of the hearing aid

_____

b. List the options on the hearing aid (telecoils or direct audio input capability?)

_____

_____

4. List any specialized equipment that is difficult to use because of the hearing loss or the hearing aids. (Computer, Stethoscope, 2-way radio, cell phone)

The goal is to identify necessary equipment that is difficult to use because of the hearing loss or the hearing aids. Knowing the level of hearing loss and hearing aid information will determine potential solutions.

For example: A nurse just received hearing aids but now has trouble using a traditional stethoscope. Specialized stethoscopes are available that will interface with different styles of hearing aids like an amplified stethoscope with headphones that allows someone with in-the-ear (ITE) hearing aids to keep them in while using the stethoscope.

List Equipment and Models

_____

_____

_____

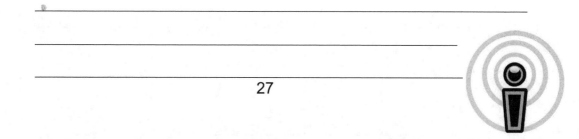

5. Obtain details about meetings.

Group listening situations are a challenge to anyone with a hearing loss and technology is available that helps in these situations. This data will determine what accommodations may be needed to make the meetings accessible, depending on the individual's preferred method of communication.

> *For example:* An individual who is late-deafened relies on captioning to follow the meeting. Schedule a CART (computer assisted real time) captionist for the monthly meetings. An interpreter is not appropriate because this individual does not know American Sign Language (ASL).

> This individual attends one meeting a week with the supervisor. Because the supervisor's office is quiet, it is not difficult to hear. However, it is difficult to hear when attending training classes several times a year with a large group (30-50 people). Here an accommodation such as CART is necessary to hear the speaker and class comments.

a. How many meetings and their frequency – describe each

_____

_____

_____

_____

_____

b. Size – how many people are in the meetings

_____

_____

_____

c. Formal and informal meetings (or video conferencing meetings)

_____

_____

d. Layout – conference table, stand around, U-shape, etc (sketch out)

```

```

6. Determine any safety issues.

The goal is to identify safety issues. These issues include equipment alarms, truck noises, fire alarms or the need to communicate while wearing hearing protection.

> *For example:* The receptionist from Step 1 has a severe hearing loss and cannot hear the fire alarm, especially in the break room where vending machines are running. The fire alarm company recommends that strobe lights be installed for the break room and bathrooms.

  a. Emergency notification – fire, etc.
      i. How is notification provided now? Is notification the same for all levels of management? (In some factories, the department level personnel use pagers to be alerted quickly.)
     ii. Does the building have an existing fire alarm system? Can strobe lights be added into the system?

_____

_____

_____

_____

b. Equipment warning sounds
    i. Do people need to hear forklift horns?
   ii. Do people need to hear alarms on any other equipment?

_____

_____

_____

_____

c. Is hearing protection required? (what type/brand is currently used?)

_____

7. Get details about phone use (and then model details in #8).

The ability to use the phone is a very common job function and is one of the easiest to accommodate. Technology is available to help almost anyone with hearing aids as well as those who rely on the relay service for visual or text communication.

> *For example:* Our receptionist from Step 1 tried using a headset to help block out some of the background noise, but the hearing aid squealed and she could not use it. She answers the phone 30+ times a day.

a. Is it necessary to answer phones in different locations?

_____

b. How many calls are made/answered a day?

_____

c. Does a headset need to be used?

_____

d. Is a cell phone used regularly?

_____

_____

8. Get details about any equipment that is used.

This technical information is required so that compatible accessories may be obtained.

For example: The telephone system is a Norstar system and it is in a newer building that has a digital phone system. Digital phone lines cannot accommodate special amplified telephones nor can they activate telephone ring signalers. The goal is to use the existing telephone so that all the features are available. If a specialty phone is needed, then the phone port must be switched to analog (the same port that a fax machine needs).

If a headset is used, find the name of the headset and the amplifier that it plugs into. You should be able to describe what the plug on the headset looks like (quick disconnect or a telephone jack). For a cell phone, you need both the model and model number (Nokia 5780).

a. Identify the model of the telephone.

_____

b. What are the models of 2-way radios and cell phones?

_____

c. Determine if the office phone system is digital or analog.

_____

d. What is the brand of headset being used by others in the office?

_____

9. Determine the issues related to travel for a person with hearing loss.

There are accommodations that can be requested in advance to make travel safe and meetings accessible. There are strategies that can make communicating with travel personnel easier. Resources are available that discuss travel issues for people with hearing loss.

For example: An employee attends a conference and must be able to use the phone in the hotel room, be awakened by the alarm clock, and must hear the phone ring. The workshops are large groups of 30 or more and it is difficult to hear the speaker. Lunch banquets or social events are especially hard because of distance from the speaker and background noise.

a. Does the employee fly or drive a great deal?

_____

b. When staying in a hotel, can the employee hear the alarm clock, fire alarm or someone knocking on door? Can he or she hear on the telephone?

_____

c. Are accommodations requested for any conferences or meetings?

_____

10. Determine the person's communication preference.

Give your employees real-time access to meetings by providing their preferred method of communication. If attendance is expected by other staff, then access should be available to the person with hearing loss. The company benefits by removing barriers to full participation and enabling the employee to work at his or her full potential.

For example: The receptionist may prefer to use her residual hearing and hearing aids to hear in meetings. An adult who is late deafened may prefer captioning during meetings for real time access.

a. Is speech the preferred method of communication?
Hard of hearing individuals may wish to use their residual hearing and hearing aids when communicating along with any assistive technology that may help.

_____

_____

_____

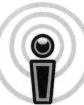

b. Is written communication desired?

Notetakers, captionists, email, text messaging and relay services may provide the most accessible means of communication.

c. Are ASL interpreters preferred?

Individuals who use sign language as their primary method of communication will expect qualified interpreters at meetings, etc.

Now what?

Now that all the issues are documented, it is time to develop a plan for accommodations. This next step requires management support, creativity and an open mind. The questions below are an excellent starting point as you look at the data gathered.

What process changes are possible?
- Change or adjust job duties.
- Challenge the status quo. The comment "It has always been done this way" is not acceptable.
- Incorporate new strategies for meetings or informal conversations.

What environmental changes can be made?
- Move or rearrange offices.
- Use carpeting and acoustic tiles in unfriendly listening environments.
- Heighten cubicle walls.
- Add mirrors and marked walkways for safety in high traffic areas.

What personnel issues should be addressed?
- Make sure all interested parties are part of the process.
- Provide top-down support to reinforce desired outcomes.
- Determine if awareness training may be helpful.
- Address behavioral issues of the employee or his or her co-workers that may impede successful accommodations.

What technology can be used to overcome a barrier?
- Identify the resources available that can assist in recommending technology.
- Work with the telecommunications and maintenance personnel for assistance in installing any technology.

The remaining chapters of this book address many of these issues in detail. I recommend that you read all the chapters if you are new to accommodating someone with a hearing loss so that you become acquainted with the many obstacles and solutions for this invisible disability.

Forms are available in the back of this book to help gather information. On-line resources that will provide up-to-date information from an employment standpoint as well as personal resources for the employee with hearing loss will are also included.

Chapter 4 – Telephone Issues

Hearing on the telephone is a critical job function for many people. The factors that contribute to using the phone successfully include environmental strategies, communication strategies and technology solutions.

Environmental Strategies

- If the person is in an open office environment and background noise is an issue, then adding fabric panel wall dividers will help reduce offending background noise.
- If the individual is behind a counter or glass panel, the use of an assistive device may be helpful because it can place a microphone closer to the person speaking.
- If the work station is next to a busy traffic area, or near metal filing cabinets, moving the workstation can improve listening on the phone.

Communication Strategies for the Phone

- Tell people how to talk to you when on the phone. Ask them to speak slower or louder so that you can hear them more clearly.
- Repeat back what you think you understood so the caller knows what you have missed. This helps to confirm understanding, especially of critical information.

Technology Solutions

Here are several tactics to use in overcoming the obstacles that hearing aids and telephones may pose. These are some of the most common problems that occur when trying to use the phone with hearing aids:

If you can't hear the caller:
The phone amplifier is the number one accommodation requested of employers. An inline phone amplifier fits in between the handset and base of most office phones and can offer 20-40 dB volume gain. A model with adjustable tone control further enhances speech understanding. Battery operated amplifiers are most popular when multiple phones are used or if electrical access is at a premium.

An inline phone amplifier will allow all the features of the phone system to remain in use. If an inline phone amplifier does not prove useful, then strong amplified phones or text phones are available. These phones are designed for home use and require an analog phone line to operate. If the phone system is digital, a port needs to be changed to analog (the same type of line as a fax machine).

If the hearing aid squeals when using the phone:

- Attach a foam earpad to the earpiece of the phone to create a space between the hearing aid and the handset. The drawback to foam pads is that the handset may not fit back into the cradle to hang up properly. Use a rubber band to secure the pad to the earpiece if you try one before adhering it permanently to the phone.

- Use the telecoil option on the hearing aid. The telecoil (or t-coil or telephone switch) is an effective way to interface the hearing aid and telephone. The telecoil helps reduce background noise and prevents or reduces squealing because it turns off the hearing aid microphone and uses an induction signal to process the sound.

- If a static or humming sound is experienced when trying to use the telecoil on the hearing aid, it may be caused by a computer CRT screen or overhead fluorescent lights. Try using an LCD monitor or different lighting to compensate.

- The other hearing aid option that can bypass the telecoil and is not susceptible to the interference is called Direct Audio Input. A cable that runs from the phone and connects directly to the hearing aid is called DAI. The audiologist should be involved if this option is explored. DAI is not an option for headset use.

If you must wear a headset: (like customer service representatives)

The first obstacle is to find a headset style that can be worn while hearing aids are in. In-the-ear style hearing aids are probably the easiest to interface headsets with. There also are leatherette pads that go over foam headsets to provide more space and sometimes help reduce squealing if feedback is an issue.

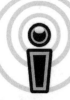

If new hearing aids are going to be purchased, it is important to bring the headset in to the hearing healthcare provider. In-the-canal style hearing aids work well with headsets. In-the-ear hearing aids sometimes cause feedback so it is important to work closely with the hearing healthcare professional. In-the-ear aids that feature a push button to operate the hearing aid can cause problems if the button is activated when headphones are placed over the ear.

Headset use becomes increasingly difficult when trying to interface with behind-the-ear style hearing aids. Traditional headsets are not adaptable to BTE hearing aids. A headset that creates an induction signal is often helpful and several styles exist to interface with cell phones, cordless phones. One common amplifier uses a special adapter cable so that an induction headset can be used.

Binaural listening (listening with both hearing aids) can often improve speech understanding when on the phone so a headset with dual earphones may be desirable. Binaural headphones also provide more protection from background noise. Monaural headsets may be a better option for receptionists or others who must use the phone and hear customers at the same time.

Usually headsets and amplifiers cannot be mixed and matched. Almost all headsets require an amplifier that fits between the handset and base of the phone and these two units must be compatible. For example, if a Plantronics amplifier is not compatible with the phone model, then Plantronics headsets cannot be used.

Headset manufacturers change models frequently so it is important to find out the current models when these issues need to be addressed.

Options to consider if the amplified phones do not help:

When all other options have been unsuccessful, it is still possible to conduct a clear conversation on the phone. Traditional relay services provide a way for individuals who are deaf or hard of hearing to engage in two-way communication. A relay operator types what the hearing caller says and then reads the text typed by the person with hearing loss back to the hearing caller.

The Telecommunications Relay Service (TRS) is a national service mandated by Title IV of the Americans with Disabilities Act of 1990.

Users can access this free service by using a TTY (or TDD) which is a text device with a display screen and keyboard that allows a person who is hard of hearing or deaf to type their end of the conversation while reading what the other party is saying. TRS is a traditional text to voice relay service.

Relay services are available in every state and the service itself is free for local calling (long distance charges will apply for long distance calls). The relay service is accessed by phone and internet. Often it is possible to dial 711 to reach the relay provider that serves the state from which the call originates. The relay number is also listed in the front of the phone book. The TRS website is listed in the Resource chapter as well as some of the other service providers for the most up-to-date information available.

Relay services provide several other ways to assist in phone conversations:

VCO (voice carry over) is a relay service that provides text of the caller's part of the conversation while allowing the deaf or hard of hearing person to use their own voice (instead of typing to the relay operator) to communicate. The relay operator types only the conversation from the hearing person. A special phone called a VCO phone is needed to display the text.

Captel (captioned telephone) service provides even faster communication. The relay operator provides the text from the hearing caller's conversation but the special phone also allows that caller's voice to come through the handset. This gives the user the ability to both listen and read the conversation at the same time.

Video relay service (VRS) is a different type of service that is important to preferred by those people who use American Sign Language (ASL) to communicate. Video relay services can be accessed by using a high-speed or broadband internet connection (DSL or T1 line) and a videophone connected to a TV, or by using video conferencing software like Microsoft NetMeeting, a computer monitor, web camera and special software.

The deaf or hard of hearing individual communicates with the relay operator who is a sign language interpreter by using the TV or monitor. The ASL user will communicate directly with the interpreter for a more natural and free flowing conversation while the interpreter

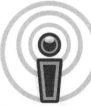

speaks to the hearing caller. VRS provides visual communication instead of text communication.

Relay and Video Relay companies are introducing new advances to the technology and services at a rapid pace. Data available today can be changed or obsolete tomorrow. It is important to review the websites in the Resource chapter for the most up-to-date information on relay services and cell phones.

If hearing on the cell phone is difficult:

Cell phones can present another challenge for hearing aid users. The ability to interface hearing aids to a cell phone is important and while more phones are now required to be hearing aid compatible, there still are difficulties. Cell phone companies are required to have available and allow testing of hearing aid compatible cell phone models.

Cell phone accessories are available to help hearing aid users interface with the cell phone by using either telecoils or direct audio input. Both of these options provide hands-free use but must be plugged into the cell phone. The disadvantage is that hearing aid users must contend with cords every time they use the phone.

Bluetooth technologies are becoming more main-stream and widely available. Bluetooth communication eliminates the cords and allows for easy use of the phone for people with and without hearing aids. The benefits of Bluetooth are open to hearing aid users who have telecoils in their hearing aids or direct audio input into their behind-the-ear hearing aids. Bluetooth technology will advance quickly now that it is becoming more common.

If you cannot hear the phone is ringing:

It is often difficult to hear or distinguish which telephone is ringing in an office. If the phone system has analog phone lines, a signaler can flash a lamp or vibrate a belt-worn receiver to alert to the phone ringing. An adjustable tone ringer is another option to help distinguish one phone ringing from another one.

There are fewer options if the phone lines are digital. Signalers often are not sensitive enough to pick up the weaker signals from digital lines. However, one option is to change the phone port to analog (something the phone company handles) so that signaler will work. Another option to try, if the office is quiet, is a sound monitor like the baby cry signaler to pick up the audible ring of the phone. The sound signaler can alert you by either flashing a lamp plugged into a remote receiver or vibrating a personal, belt-worn receiver.

In Conclusion

The technology exists to help with telephone solutions, but it changes at a rapid pace. If you understand the potential solutions, use Chapter 11 to provide resources that will point you to the most up-to-date information available.

Chapter 5 – Mastering Meetings

Meetings are perhaps the most unpopular job functions for people with hearing loss. Many people with hearing loss stop attending meetings and rely on co-workers or managers to 'fill them in'. Others bravely attempt the meeting only to sit quietly without fully participating. However, there are consequences for not participating in real time.

Issues for an Employer to Consider

If an employer provides training opportunities or expects staff to participate in meetings, then providing accommodations is reasonable. A person with hearing loss is hindered without appropriate accommodations. By incorporating the techniques listed in this chapter, an employer can also ensure accessible meetings for employees with and without hearing loss.

One-on-one meetings with a supervisor in an office are the easiest to maneuver for people with most any level of hearing loss because the office is typically quiet and there are no distractions. Communication is at its best in this situation.

The most common threats to clear communication in meetings are multiple speakers, distance from the speaker and background noise. While an employee may be able to plan for scheduled meetings, informal meetings are probably the hardest to anticipate and may be the hardest to accommodate.

Often, meetings consist of multiple speakers in active conversation. This is especially true in heated discussions or brainstorming sessions. It is difficult for a person with hearing loss to follow these conversations. It can be nearly impossible to keep up while trying to identify who is speaking.

Distance from the speaker makes it difficult to hear clearly. Sound waves lose intensity only a few feet from the speaker. If the speaker does not project his or her voice well, those people towards the back of the room will always have difficulty hearing.

Background noise can cause interference during a meeting. It can come from side conversations while the main speaker is talking. It may come when the air conditioning system kicks on and creates a constant humming sound that can be disastrous to a person wearing hearing aids.

A doomed meeting

Jan has called an impromptu meeting for the team. There are windows on one side of the room and Jan leads the meeting while sitting in front of those windows. Jan did not prepare an agenda so discussion skips from one topic to another. People sometimes talk over one another or it seems that one team member dominates the meeting. No one wrote summary notes on an overhead or board and the meeting only stops because it is the end of the day.

It is easy to use basic meeting etiquette to turn that same meeting into a success for everyone. Meeting etiquette can improve every meeting. Some may feel that following meeting rules will squash the spontaneity. But a few moments for advance preparations can lead to successful meetings.

A moderator or facilitator is assigned at the beginning of the meeting and his or her role is explained: Keep the meeting running on schedule, break a discussion if necessary and remind people of the rules.

Meeting Manners

- Prepare an agenda and stick to it – use graphics when appropriate
- Make the outcome of the meeting clear
- Choose a time when the meeting will end
- Assign a moderator or facilitator to help keep meeting rules
- Set meeting rules
    - One person speaks at a time
    - Don't start another topic until the current topic is closed
    - Use a microphone if necessary
- Consider the meeting room layout and rearrange as necessary
- Schedule a note-taker or interpreter
    - Secure an assistive listening device
    - Wrap up the meeting with a summary

Issues for an Employee to Consider

Many people with hearing loss report that they do not participate in meetings because it is so difficult to keep up. It is embarrassing to say something that has already been said or offer a comment on a subject, only to find that the subject has already changed. Using the strategies outlined here may help improve this difficult situation.

Job performance can be adversely affected when someone doesn't participate in meetings. Not participating is perceived as not caring or not being 'part of the team.' Enlisting the help of a coworker or manager to follow meeting etiquette manners makes it easier to participate.

Conferences or Training Meetings:

Conference workshops are challenging. It is important to request accommodations in advance, such as interpreters, CART reporting or FM systems. It is helpful to get to the workshop early enough to find the most favorable seating. If an FM system is used, it might be helpful to talk with the presenter in advance and ask them to repeat any questions from the attendees before answering them.

Luncheon and dinner banquets are difficult. There is often a presentation during the banquet as well as free time to talk with others at the table. Tables usually seat 8-10 people and conversations with those seated nearby will be easy while hearing across the table may be exasperating. The same accommodations for the workshops can be used for any general meetings/banquets, etc.

Social events are the most difficult to maneuver because of larger crowds or background music (noise). The use of an FM system is very effective in these situations if one is comfortable using it.

If you are the speaker, there are strategies you can use to ease communication issues. First, enlist help from meeting planners/volunteers for any help you need. It may be as simple as asking someone in the audience to use an FM system to repeat questions so that you may hear clearly.

Set rules at the beginning of the presentation. Instruct people to raise their hands to ask a question, or stand up when asking the question so that you can speechread better. Use a stand-alone microphone or pass the microphone for an assistive listening system.

If you are the audience member, there are steps you can take to improve this very difficult listening situation.

Environmental Strategies

- If the speaker is in front of the room, plan to arrive early for more favorable seating.
- Sit at round tables or move tables into a square whenever possible. This gives you the ability to see everyone's face.
- When sitting in a U-shape, sit close to the primary speaker. You will be able to see others around the table.
- Sit facing away from any windows in the room or close the blinds. It is difficult to see someone who is speaking in front of a window.
- If you can't hear everyone, ask to switch seats for better listening.
- If air-conditioning or blowers are loud, arrange to meet in a different area for future meetings.

Communication Strategies

Use Good Meeting Rules

- Distribute written agendas in advance.
- Appoint one person as the meeting facilitator.
- Allow only one person to speak at a time.
- Plan for good visuals when appropriate.
- Insist speakers use the PA system microphone when available.
- Use an assistive listening system and pass the microphone (or try a conference microphone.)
- Arrange for an interpreter or CART reporting before the meeting

Technology Solutions

- Seek advice from a hearing healthcare provider if you don't have hearing aids.

- Use an assistive listening system. Assistive listening systems are designed specifically to improve the speech signal and reduce background noise by placing the microphone close to the desired sound source. These systems can be used with or without hearing aids. See the Resources chapter for more information.

- Use computer assisted note-taking or Computer Assisted Real-Time Captioning (CART) or an interpreter. These services are available remotely. See the Resources chapter for more information on these services.

Exploring the potential solutions offered here will enhance the process and help everyone stay on track, hear more clearly and participate more fully. Success depends on the ability to be assertive when requesting or using these accommodations.

Chapter 6 – Blasting Background Noise

The world is a noisy place. Noise can be a simple nuisance or it can become an uncompromising obstacle. Background noise can plague a hearing aid wearer in situations that normal hearing people never notice.

The number one complaint of people who wear hearing aids is the inability to understand speech in background noise. The ability to hear when background noise is present can adversely affect job performance. This chapter is devoted to some creative ways to communicate in these 'unfriendly' environments.

A variety of products will help improve speech understanding when background noise is present. The goal is to increase the so-called signal-to-noise ratio (SNR) by increasing the volume of the desired sound without increasing the level of noise.

Unfriendly Communication Situations

Certain listening situations and environments are always difficult because of background noise or reverberation. Reverberation is a problem in large rooms, cafeterias and gymnasiums where the sounds bounce off the hard reflective walls and floors.

Typical Job Situations

- Factory Work
- Open floor plans in offices
- Large or very busy offices
- Outdoor work (car salespeople, construction, law enforcement where communication demands are high with customers, coworkers and the public)
- Cafeteria/lunchrooms
- Luncheons, restaurants, social situations

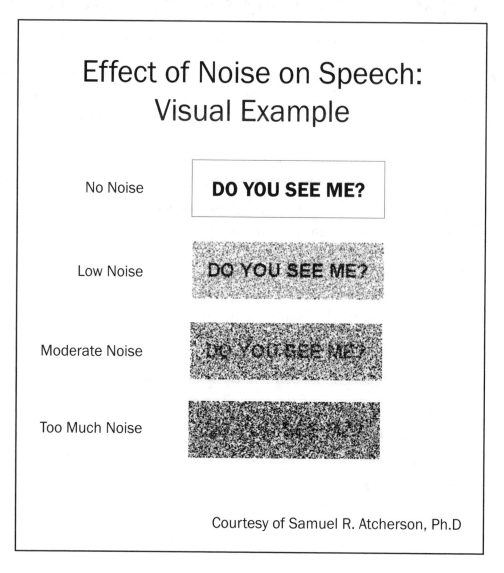

Effect of Noise on Speech: Visual Example

No Noise — **DO YOU SEE ME?**

Low Noise — DO YOU SEE ME?

Moderate Noise — DO YOU SEE ME?

Too Much Noise —

Courtesy of Samuel R. Atcherson, Ph.D

As the level of background noise increases, the speech signal becomes weaker and more distorted. The ultimate goal is to increase the speech signal so that speech remains clear even in competing noise. Technology solutions to this dilemma are discussed in Chapter 9, Technical Solution #2, Assistive Listening Systems.

Issues to Consider

There are several issues to consider when analyzing background noise and its impact on the ability to communicate. As the employee, it is important to be as specific as possible as you identify these situations:

- What are the specific communication demands with coworkers and customers?

- What sounds specifically interfere with these communication situations? (machinery, fans, large number of people, copiers, general outdoor noise)

- What style of hearing instruments is being used?

- Is hearing protection required?

- Are there safety issues to be addressed?

Possible Solutions

There are basically three ways to improve communication when background noise is present:

1. **Control the environment as much as possible.** Find a quieter area for essential communication when necessary. Consider moving your workspace to a quieter area, or placing your back to the noise. Move away from copy machines or fans. Request cubicle walls to reduce noise. Eliminate white noise filters in open areas. Use an assistive listening system when communicating with clients or customers. Make sure essential communication occurs in a quieter location.

2. **Talk with your hearing health care provider** and describe your work and social situations. Hearing instruments with directional microphones may help in noisy situations when you are facing the person you need to speak with. Programmable hearing instruments may allow your hearing aid to perform more effectively when noise is present. The need to wear hearing protection may determine the type of hearing instrument you need. The telecoil is a hearing aid option that allows you to interface most effectively and discreetly with an assistive listening system.

3. **Use an assistive listening system** when communicating with customers and co-workers. An assistive listening system like an FM system is designed specifically to improve the speech signal and reduce background noise by placing the microphone close to the desired sound source.

Overcoming the communication challenges when background noise is present is one area where the combination of hearing instruments, communication strategies and assistive technology can provide significant improvement.

Case Studies
Solutions to communicating when background noise is present.

Jason, a car salesperson, asks customers to wear an FM transmitter with a lapel microphone while walking through the car lot. He uses the receiver with a neckloop and turns one hearing aid onto telecoil. Now he can remain aware of environmental sounds while also hearing the customer more clearly. He is a more effective salesperson when he can appropriately respond to questions and concerns.

Mike, a factory worker, uses a hearing protection headset that has microphones on the ear cups. He simply turns on the microphones to hear the person in front of him. When finished, he turns off the headset to resume full hearing protection.

Marion cannot tell when her phone is ringing in a large busy office. She uses a visual alerting device connected to the phone and mounted up on the wall.

Mike, the factory worker, cannot hear overhead pages. The company uses a paging system similar to those used in restaurants. The company placed the base transmitter on the receptionist desk. Any time Mike must be alerted to a page, the receptionist enters 3 numbers and presses TRANSMIT. Mike wears a vibrating receiver with an LCD numeric display (0-9). The codes are preset to specific messages. For example, 9=emergency or fire, 0=go the front desk, 1=go to the loading dock, etc. He knows where to go based on the code.

Chapter 7 – Non-Technical Solutions

Environmental changes, procedural changes and communication strategies can improve a work environment before adding additional technology. These solutions are often the most important to implement because they may change the need for any technical solutions.

Process changes or job duty changes can improve overall performance.

- Adjust or change job duties.
- Challenge the status quo. The comment "It has always been done this way" is not acceptable.
- Incorporate new strategies for meetings or informal conversations.

Environmental changes often eliminate or reduce communication challenges.

- Move or rearrange offices.
- Use carpeting and acoustic tiles in unfriendly listening environments.
- Heighten cubicle walls.
- Add mirrors and marked walkways for safety in high traffic areas.

Non technical solutions include team support

- Make sure all interested parties are part of the process.
- Provide top-down support to reinforce desired outcomes.
- Determine if awareness training may be helpful.
- Address behavioral issues of the employee or his or her co-workers that are impeding successful accommodations.

Dr. Trychin's **Living With Hearing Loss Program** is a product of twenty-two years of experience working directly with hundreds of people who are hard of hearing and their family members. Additionally, many more people who are hard of hearing, their family members, and professionals who serve them have benefited from his training programs, presentations, and workshops.

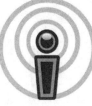

Hearing loss is a communication disorder affecting everyone in the communication situation-- the person speaking as well as the person with hearing loss who is trying to listen. For that reason, the *Living With Hearing Loss Program* is designed to meet the needs of family members, friends, coworkers, and service providers as well as the person who is hard of hearing. The overall focus is on helping people:

- Manage themselves--by reducing the physical/emotional/cognitive distress related to hearing loss.

- Manage situations--by preventing and reducing communication and other problems related to hearing loss.

The **Kooser Program** is an aural rehabilitation program used by vocational rehabilitation agencies and audiology groups to improve the quality of life of persons with hearing loss by empowerment through education and support services.

The program is 12 hours in length and seeks to educate the person with hearing loss as well as their loved ones regarding the psychosocial impact of this disability. It teaches positive coping skills and communication strategies, as well as discusses many pertinent issues including hearing loss in the workplace, assertive behavior, the grief process and how it impacts relationships.

Common Communication Tips

Tips for Speaking to a Person with Hearing Loss

- Reduce or move the conversation away from background noise.
- Wait until the person with hearing loss can see you before speaking.
- Speak at a normal tempo. This will aid in speech-reading.
- Be aware of your voice modulation. A very loud voice that is further amplified by a hearing aid can be distressing and sometimes painful to the wearer.
- If a person seems to hear but does not understand you, shouting will not help. It is also wise not to drop the volume of your voice at the end of a sentence.

- Repeat your statement if it is not understood and then try to rephrase it.

- Enunciate well without distorting your speech. Remember that the listener may not understand all words even when they are properly articulated. Consonants can be particularly difficult to understand. Some pairs of letters frequently cause confusion – examples include meet vs. beet, shoe vs. chew and few vs. view.

- Avoid chewing or covering your mouth. Keep your hands away from your mouth while speaking.

- Clue the person to any changes in the discussion topic. Doing so may involve using several different words to express the same thought.

- Be patient.

Tips for a Person with Hearing Loss

- Do not bluff.

- Reduce or move the conversation away from background noise.

- Confirm and verify. Repeat what you heard for confirmation.

- Anticipate typical communication situations such as drive-through services or waiters at restaurants.

- Be patient and add humor.

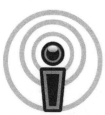

Chapter 8 – Technical Solution #1
Hearing Aid Solutions

This chapter is devoted to helping you understand how hearing aids and cochlear implants work in general. As an employer, you don't need to know all the technical details about hearing aids so we are going to focus on the features that you do need to know.

Individuals with hearing loss will want to know more about the types of hearing aids and should educate themselves on what technology is currently available. Although this type of information is not covered in this book, resources are listed in Chapter 12.

Assistive listening systems, specifically FM systems, have different listening options based on the hearing aid and level of hearing loss. The ability to interface an assistive listening system to a hearing aid is vitally important for effective communication. You'll learn how hearing aids interface to FM systems and other assistive listening systems.

- Hearing Aid basics
- Cochlear Implant Basics
- Hearing Aid Styles
- Hearing Aid/Cochlear Implant Options

Hearing Aid Basics

Hearing aid technology has come a long way from the hearing aids of even 5 years ago. Improvements in circuit miniaturization and advancements in digital processing provide more natural sounds and improved clarity.

Hearing aids are dispensed by a hearing healthcare professional (audiologist or hearing instrument specialist). They will assess the level of hearing loss and the communication needs of the individual. They will then recommend the style and options of the most appropriate hearing aids.

Hearing aids don't correct hearing loss and it is reasonable to expect follow-up visits to the dispenser in order for adjustments to be made that will provide optimum performance of the aids. This is especially true if someone works in an 'unfriendly listening environment'. The challenges from demanding communication situations may require additional fine-tuning as well.

Cochlear Implant Basics

A cochlear implant is another hearing technology. It is a medical device that consists of two parts. One part is the internal electrode component that is surgically implanted into the inner ear (cochlea) to bypass damaged hair cells. The electrode array will directly stimulate the hearing nerve.

The external part of the system is called the speech processor. It looks similar to a behind-the-ear hearing aid. The processor digitizes sound and codes the signal to transmit to the internal part of the system. Some speech processors are body worn processors instead of ear level. Direct audio input and telecoil are available on most speech processors.

There is also basic information about hearing loss, hearing aids and cochlear implants that must be known in order to help accommodate an individual with hearing loss. These facts will determine how the hearing aid will be able to interface with any type of assistive listening system or amplified telephone. You won't be able to dispense hearing aids after reading this, but you will know the terminology of the data you will gather.

You will need the following information:

- Level of hearing loss (an audiogram is good to have if possible).
- Style of the hearing aid or cochlear implant.
- Options of the hearing aid.

Hearing Aid Styles

There are three major types of hearing aid styles:

- CIC
- ITE
- BTE

Completely-In-The-Canal Hearing Aid (CIC)

CIC hearing aids are very small and discreet. They are too small to add options like a telecoil. However, the telecoil may not be needed as long as phone use can be accomplished without squealing (or feedback). One major consideration for this style of hearing aid is the size of the ear canal. The ear canal may not be large enough to accommodate a CIC aid. CIC aids are typically intended for mild to moderate hearing loss.

CIC hearing aids are a viable option for certain occupations and the hearing professional will be able to determine this. This style hearing aid must be able to interface to telephones and perhaps an assistive listening system via headphones.

Custom In-The-Ear Hearing Aids (ITE)

ITE hearing aids are probably the most common hearing aid on the market and are typically intended for mild to severe degrees of hearing loss. ITE aids come in a range of sizes from very small in-the-canal aids to those that fill the bowl of the ear entirely, also known as full shell aids. These aids may have telecoils.

ITE hearing aids must be able to interface to telephones without squealing (or feedback). If listening situations with background noise are present, the inclusion of a telecoil will be helpful for interfacing to assistive listening systems.

Behind-The-Ear Hearing Aids (BTE) or Cochlear Implants

The BTE hearing aid sits behind the ear and is attached to a custom made earmold that fits in the ear. BTE hearing aids can be fit to every type of hearing loss. They vary in size depending on the circuitry and amplification requirements. These aids may have telecoils and the option for direct audio input.

Cochlear Implant speech processors are now shaped like a behind-the-ear hearing aid and may include a telecoil option and direct audio input capability.

If telephone use is a primary job function, then telecoils are desired so that an effective interface to an amplified telephone or assistive listening system is present. Telephone headset use is not normally effective with behind-the-ear style hearing aids, especially if the individual has a more severe hearing loss.

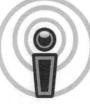

Hearing Aid/Cochlear Implant Optional Features

Hearing aids and cochlear implants come with a variety of optional features:

Telephone switch (t-coil or telecoil)

The purpose of a telecoil is to bypass the hearing aid microphone to obtain a sound signal. If a hearing aid squeals when trying to use a telephone, the only way to stop the feedback is to remove the hearing aid or turn the microphone down. This is not an effective option for anyone with a more severe hearing loss.

The telecoil is a small coiled wire placed within the hearing aid designed to pick up an induction signal from an audio source. The telecoil allows the hearing aid to process sound differently without the hearing aid microphone. Now the individual gets the full benefit of the hearing aid that has been programmed for his or her hearing loss.

The telecoil is activated usually with a switch on the hearing aid. Some hearing aids have an auto-telecoil that only activates when the phone is placed next to the hearing aid. This is an excellent option for someone who is on the phone all day, but it is a bad option if one wants to use an assistive listening system.

Cochlear implants either have the telecoil built into the speech processor or an attachment is placed on the processor to provide a telecoil interface.

Direct Audio Input (DAI)

Direct audio input refers to a direct electrical connection from the audio source directly to the hearing aid. DAI is available on most behind-the-ear hearing aids. It is not an option for in-the-ear hearing aids. An audio shoe snaps onto the hearing aid case and makes a direct connection. The audio shoe will accept a cable or receiver that plugs into it.

Direct audio input is also available for cochlear implants. There are accessories usually included in the cochlear implant for direct audio connection.

Volume control wheel

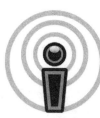

Most hearing aids have a wheel that can be turned to increase the amplification. Depending on the age and style of hearing aid, the telecoil may perform better if the volume control is turned up and subsequently turned back down when leaving the aid on the microphone setting.

Programmable aids may be best for multiple listening environments because many feature multiple memories. For example, one for conversations in quiet and another for conversations in noisy places like a restaurant. The programs may be accessed either with a remote control or with a button on the hearing aid.

The Relation of Hearing Aids, Hearing Aid Options and ALD Listening Options

Hearing aids can provide tremendous benefit in most all general listening situations. The ability to interface the hearing aid with an assistive listening system (or ALD) in difficult listening environments can maximize the benefit and performance of the hearing aid. An FM system is an assistive listening system.

Understanding the relation of hearing aids, hearing aid options and ALD listening options can help improve the successful use of an ALD and increased communication ability.

Chapter 9 - Technical Solution #2
Assistive Listening Systems (Specifically FM Systems)

Assistive listening systems, specifically FM systems, have different listening options based on the hearing aid and level of hearing loss. The ability to interface an assistive listening system to a hearing aid is vitally important for effective communication. The goal of this chapter is to help you learn how hearing aids interface to FM systems and other assistive listening systems.

There are three types of assistive listening systems that transmit sound from a microphone to a personal listening device. Each one uses a different type of transmission:

• FM systems use special radio frequencies to transmit sound.
• Infrared systems use infrared light beams to transmit sound.
• Loop systems create an induction signal to transmit sound to hearing aids with telecoils.

All three of these systems perform basically the same function. They are designed to overcome distance from the speaker and unfavorable listening conditions such as room acoustics and reverberation by placing a microphone close to the sound source. They deliver the sound to the ear (or hearing aid) and produce a clear sound signal.

How does an FM System Work?

Room acoustics, background noise and distance from the speaker will affect the speech signal by reducing the intensity and clarity of speech. By the time the hearing aid microphone picks up the sound signal, the sound signal is corrupted.

An FM system consists of two units, a transmitter and receiver. The transmitter is equipped with a microphone that is clipped to the lapel of the speaker. It transmits sound using radio frequency to the other unit, called a receiver. The receiver is worn by the person with hearing loss. It is equipped with an appropriate listening option to interface with the hearing aid or cochlear implant.

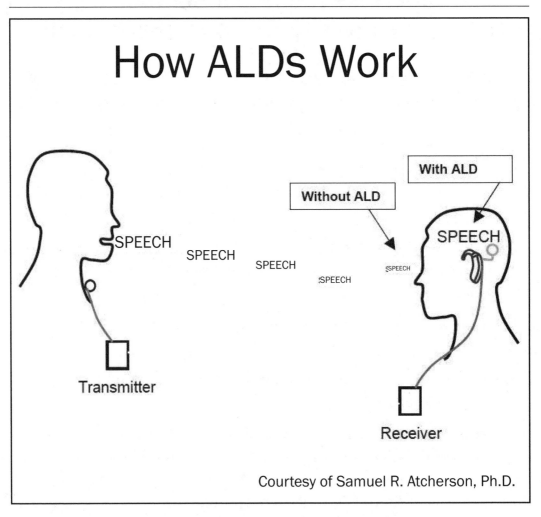

How ALDs Work

With ALD

Without ALD

SPEECH

SPEECH

SPEECH

SPEECH

SPEECH

SPEECH

Transmitter

Receiver

Courtesy of Samuel R. Atcherson, Ph.D.

Hearing Aid Styles and Listening Options

CICs/ITCs: Very small instruments that fit completely in the canal or deep in the canal. ALD listening options: headphones or earphone.

ITEs: Instruments that fit in-the-ear and may fill the bowl of the ear. ITE aids generally have room for a telecoil. It is a special circuit in the hearing aid that allows the person to use the full power of their hearing aid without feedback. ALD listening options: earphone, neckloop or silhouette.

BTEs: Instruments with an ear mold that fits in the ear and attaches to the aid behind the ear. BTE aids have several optional features that provide effective interfaces (telecoil and direct audio input).

When using BTE aids, snap on wireless receivers can replace one of the components of the traditional FM system. ALD listening options: neckloop, silhouette, patch cord, snap-on wireless receiver, Bluetooth device (maybe some headphones or earphones).

Cochlear Implants: Many speech processors have both the telecoil and direct audio input options available. ALD listening options: neckloop, silhouette, patch cord, snap-on wireless receiver, Bluetooth device (maybe some headphones).

How to Interface to the FM System without Hearing Aids

FM Listening Options: Without Hearing Aids

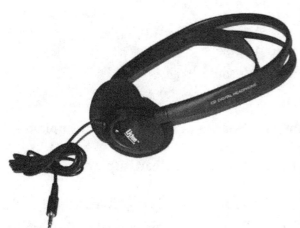

Headphones: Standard headphones that fit over the head (or behind the head). Headphones are for mild to moderate loss. They provide sound to both ears and may be the most effective if a person must listen for a long period of time. They may cause feedback and sound leakage at higher volume levels because the headphones do not fit tight over the ear. This sound leakage could cause distraction to others.

Earphone: Basically half a headphone that fits over one ear with an adjustable hook. It is more appealing to many because it is more discreet but only delivers sound to one ear. Earphones are designed for mild to moderate hearing losses. The single earphone allows 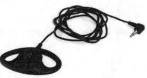 one ear to receive the sound signal while the other ear can still hear room sounds. The earphone may cause feedback and sound leakage at high volume levels because it does not fit tight over the ear. This sound leakage could be distracting to others.

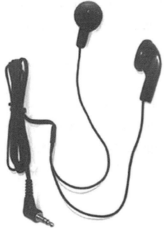

Single or Dual Earbuds: A small metal disc (usually covered with soft material) that fits snugly in the ear. Earbuds are a great listening option for individuals with more severe hearing losses because they provide a tight seal that increases the sound pressure in the ear canal. Because it's easier to hear using both ears rather than just one, dual earbuds are an even better choice.

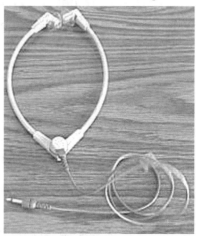

Underchin Stetoclip Headset: Looks like a stethoscope. The stetoclip headset has mushroom tips that provide an even tighter seal than dual earbuds in the ear canal. Stetoclip headsets offer great sound quality for more severe losses.

How to Interface to the FM System with Hearing Aids or Cochlear Implants

FM Listening Options with Hearing Aids and Cochlear Implants

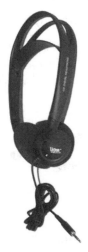

Headphones: Deliver sound to CICs. It is possible to use headphones with some ITEs or BTEs. However, squealing is usually a problem. They may cause feedback (squealing) and sound leakage at higher volume levels. This sound leakage can be distracting to others.

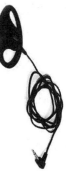

Earphone: Delivers sound to CICs and most ITEs and BTEs. They may cause feedback (squealing) and sound leakage at high volume levels. This sound leakage can be distracting to others.

Neckloops are for moderate to severe hearing loss. They can only be used with ITE or BTE hearing aids with the telecoil option. This is effective for people with more severe loss because it bypasses the hearing aid microphone, eliminating the possibility of feedback or sound leakage. This also allows for binaural listening.

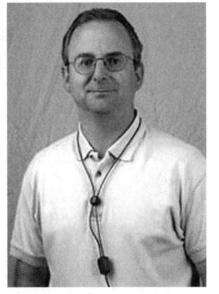

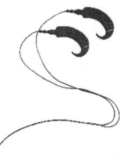

Silhouettes are also for moderate to severe hearing loss. They can only be used with ITE or BTE hearing aids with the telecoil option. Silhouettes are similar to the neckloop except the induction signal created by the silhouette is now directly next to the hearing aid's telecoil for a strong signal.

Direct audio input (DAI): Provides the cleanest signal to the hearing aid because it is a direct electrical connection. DAI allows the hearing aid microphone to remain on while also picking up the FM system signal. DAI is used for severe to profound hearing losses when:

- The telecoils are not strong enough
- The FM system is not strong enough to power a neckloop
- There is static on the telecoil setting

BTE Hearing Aid

Audio Boot

FM Wireless Receiver

If the hearing aid has DAI capability, purchase an audio shoe or boot from the hearing healthcare provider and snap it onto the BTE hearing aid to create an electrical connection between the hearing aid and either a cable or wireless FM receiver or Bluetooth receiver.

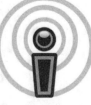

The audio shoe accepts a 3 prong standard Euro connection. FM and Bluetooth receivers have this Euro connection. Special cables also have this connection. The cable runs from the audio shoe to the FM system receiver (or other audio source).

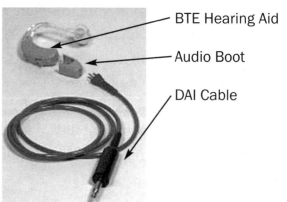

BTE Hearing Aid

Audio Boot

DAI Cable

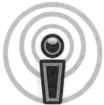

Chapter 10 – Occupations A to Z

Occupations below are grouped according to typical job functions. Many occupations share common communication challenges. If your occupation isn't listed, review the communication challenges on each report for comparisons.

- Bank Clerks
- Bus Drivers (van drivers, taxi drivers)
- Call Center Operators
- Corrections Officers
- Factory Workers (on the line or management)
- Food Service Workers (schools, cafeterias, restaurants)
- Home Health Care Personnel (CNAs, case managers, care managers, therapists, RNs)
- Inside Services and Salespersons (insurance, real estate, accounting/bookkeeping)
- Maintenance Personnel (janitorial, electrical, housekeeping)
- Managers (in an office setting or retail setting)
- Medical Professionals (vets, doctors, nurses, medical technicians in an office or medical facility)
- Office Personnel
- Outdoor Workers (construction workers, equipment operators, farmers)
- Pastors
- Retail Workers (on the floor, at the cash register or service desk)
- Teachers (instructors, meeting speakers)
- Truck Drivers

ON THE JOB WITH HEARING LOSS
Hearing Loss Issues and Bank Clerks

The purpose of this report is to help you more fully identify potential communication barriers on the job. Each report focuses on a specific employment situation or topic and offers possible solutions to typical job functions. The combination of hearing instruments, assistive technology and communication strategies play a significant role in obtaining successful communication.

Bank Clerks

Communication Demands of Typical Job Functions

- Communicate with walk-in customers
- Hear drive-through customers
- Hear on the telephone
- Communicate with co-workers in a somewhat quiet environment
- Participate in meetings

Issues to Consider and Potential Accommodations

Hearing customers from across the counter may be difficult for some people with hearing loss, especially if the person they are speaking with has a quiet voice. There are several options depending on the individual's speech discrimination. One option is to use an FM system with the transmitter microphone standing on the counter facing customers. Another option for telecoil users is the portable InfoLoop. This device would sit out on the counter facing towards customers. It has a built-in microphone and transmits an induction signal to the hearing aid telecoils wirelessly.

Hearing co-workers is important. If the individual uses either of the options above with the hearing aid set on telecoil, they will not be able to hear co-workers because the hearing aid microphone turns off when the telecoil is turned on. If it is possible to have an M/T switch (microphone + telecoil) on the hearing aid, then he or she will hear both environmental sounds plus the sound coming through the assistive listening system. Another option is to keep one hearing aid on telecoil and the other one on microphone.

Hearing drive-through customers can be challenging, especially if the speaker system is not high quality. There are many different models of radio systems and because 2-way communication is necessary, traditional style listening options for FM systems are not compatible interfaces.

Hearing conversations on the phone may easily be solved by trying an inline amplifier that fits between the handset and base of the telephone. This device provides both amplification and a stronger induction signal.

Participating in meetings is important. If the individual must attend meetings and has difficulty participating, there are options for managing meetings more efficiently. Refer to Chapter 6, Mastering Meetings for strategies and technology that can be helpful.

Hearing soft-spoken customers can be a challenge. A person with hearing loss may be able to understand one-on-one conversations at near normal conversational levels but encounter problems when trying to understand soft-spoken customers. Hearing aids provide significant hearing enhancement in this listening situation.

A personal listening system may also be helpful. See Chapter 9 for information on how to choose the right listening interface. A personal listening system allows a microphone to be placed closer to the speaker creating a better sound signal.

Case Study

Jane is a bank teller and has a moderate hearing loss. She does not currently wear hearing aids. Jane works behind the counter when customers come into the bank. She can understand most people but sometimes struggles to hear soft-spoken customers or customers with accents.

Jane also has difficulty hearing her co-workers when they talk to her. Jane must interact with drive-through customers.

Jane's hearing healthcare provider recommends in-the-ear hearing aids with telecoils and directional microphones. Jane is now able to hear co-workers and drive-through customers. She sometimes has difficulty with soft spoken customers from across the counter and has placed an FM transmitter with microphone on the counter so that the microphone is closer to the customer and she is able to hear them more clearly.

Common Technical Accommodations

- Hearing aids are the primary technology solution

- InfoLoop Portable Listening system for hearing aids with telecoils

- Inline phone amplifier

- FM system with a transmitter/microphone and a receiver with a listening option that gets the sound to the hearing aid or to the ear

ON THE JOB WITH HEARING LOSS

Hearing Loss Issues and Bus Drivers

The purpose of this report is to help you more fully identify potential communication barriers on the job. Each report focuses on a specific employment situation or topic and offers possible solutions to typical job functions. The combination of hearing instruments, assistive technology and communication strategies play a significant role in obtaining successful communication.

Bus Drivers

Bus drivers, taxi drivers and van drivers with hearing loss have several communication obstacles to address. They must be able to hear conversations from passengers while also listening to the company radio or phone, all in the presence of background noise.

Communication Demands of Typical Job Functions

- Hear passengers as they enter the vehicle
- Hear comments from passengers behind them
- Communicate with the dispatcher via radio or cellular phone
- Attend company meetings

Issues to Consider

The most effective hearing instrument can offer significant improvement. The hearing instrument must be able to interface to an assistive listening system and the radio. Directional microphones are not particularly helpful since the driver must be aware of sound both on the left and right of them as well as behind them.

Severe hearing loss and unilateral hearing loss both pose challenges in this occupation. The use of an assistive listening device becomes more important and has been a somewhat successful accommodation.

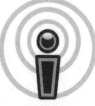

The driver must be aware of the noise surrounding him or her while also trying to listen to passengers. It is safer to keep both hearing aids turned on the microphone setting. If an FM system is to be used, then there must be an effective way of getting sound to the hearing aid.

An FM system is helpful because the transmitter with microphone can be placed close to a person boarding the bus and speaking to the driver or placed next to the radio speaker. The desired sound is louder and cleaner because the microphone is placed nearer the sound.

The FM receiver must get the sound to the hearing aid. One option is to use a neckloop that will transmit the sound to the hearing aid's telecoil. Another option on a hearing aid is an M/T switch. When set on M/T, both the hearing aid microphone and the telecoil are on at the same time.

When both the microphone and telecoil remain on at the same time, the telecoil will pick up sounds transmitted from the FM transmitter/microphone (that is placed close to the person speaking) while the hearing aid microphone picks up all the environmental sounds. The driver can switch to telecoil only if someone is speaking through the microphone of the FM system and the background is too loud to hear clearly.

Other ways to get the sound from the FM system receiver to the driver:

People with mild to moderate loss (and in-the-canal aids) may be able to use lightweight headphones or a single earphone to direct the sound to their ear. However, people with more severe hearing loss may find that the hearing aid squeals when the listening option is placed next to the hearing aid.

People with moderate to severe hearing loss who have telecoils (but no M/T switch) can get sound from an FM system and also hear environmental sounds. They can do this by leaving one hearing aid on telecoil and the other one on microphone.

People with severe loss (and behind the ear aids) will benefit more from direct audio input. Direct audio input will give them the ability to hear all sounds while also receiving sound from the FM system. These options can be discussed with the hearing healthcare provider.

Van Drivers and Taxi Drivers may benefit from an FM system. The microphone placement may be somewhat different for van drivers. They may fasten the FM transmitter and microphone to the middle of the van on a window or the ceiling. This way they can pick up the conversation from passengers. Taxi drivers may just place the FM transmitter microphone under the headrest facing towards the passenger.

The use of a loop system can also be used in the vehicle if the individual has hearing aids with an M/T switch to allow them to hear sound through the hearing aid microphone as well as through the sound signal from an assistive listening system.

This FM system can also be used at company meetings.

A note about fastening the units:

Some FM systems come in a cloth carrying pouch. The pouch can be fastened to the bus wall, window or vinyl with Velcro. Some people have created their own pouch if none is included. The purpose is to make the FM system readily available and easy to remove at the end of the day. The microphone should not be fastened directly to the window because it will pick up road noise. It is better to clip the microphone to the headrest or headliner.

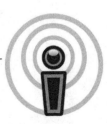

Case Study

Verna is a school bus driver with severe hearing loss. She must monitor the sounds from the bus, understand children who board the bus, hear the bus monitor and also listen to the bus radio.

Verna has a hard time understanding someone who is speaking to her when they board the bus. She must hear them but also hear the sounds from the other passengers. She has a hard time hearing the bus monitor.

An FM system transmitter with lapel microphone was used by the bus monitor. Verna wore the FM receiver and used a neckloop to get sound to her ears. Verna's receiver also had a microphone so that she could monitor sounds closer to her, approximately within arm's reach.

If a student said something as they boarded the bus and she couldn't hear them, she would hold out the receiver/microphone unit so that the sound being amplified was the child speaking to her. The bus monitor wore the FM transmitter and spoke into the lapel microphone. Verna could hear everything the bus monitor said.

If Verna had a hearing aid with M/T switch, she could turn it on and get both sounds at the same time (the bus monitor and the child speaking to her). But since her aid did not have the M/T switch, she used one aid on T (telecoil) only to pick up sounds through the FM system. The other hearing aid stayed on microphone to monitor all sounds on the bus.

Verna would often know that someone was speaking on the radio but couldn't understand them clearly. Now she reaches up and switches both aids to telecoil and asks the person to repeat. Now she gets a clean sound signal because the FM system microphone is next to the radio speaker.

This is a challenging listening environment and the FM system has been of some limited help. Verna uses the system at meetings while her supervisor wears the transmitter with microphone. She can now hear more clearly, regardless of the meeting location.

Common Technical Accommodations

- FM system with a transmitter/microphone and a receiver with environmental microphone with a listening option that gets the sound to the hearing aid or to the ear
  - Portable Microloop system installed in the vehicle

ON THE JOB WITH HEARING LOSS
Hearing Loss Issues and Call Center Operators

The purpose of this report is to help you more fully identify potential communication barriers on the job. Each report focuses on a specific employment situation or topic and offers possible solutions to typical job functions. The combination of hearing instruments, assistive technology and communication strategies play a significant role in obtaining successful communication.

Call Center Operators

Accommodating an employee with a hearing loss in a call center environment can be challenging. There are several factors to consider that can help provide an effective accommodation. One factor is the compatibility between the computer/phone system and the headset. Another factor is a compatible interface between the headset and the hearing aid.

Communication Demands of Typical Job Functions

- Interface hearing aids to the headset
- Hear callers on the phone
- Hear when background noise is present
- Complete calls in a timely manner

Issues to Consider

Summary on hearing aids

There are several styles of hearing aids. In-the-ear hearing aids may be very small and placed down in the ear canal or may be larger and fill the bowl of the ear. Behind-the-ear hearing aids wrap around to an earmold that is in the ear.

The hearing aid has a microphone. It may have a telecoil option. This is also referred to as a telephone switch. The telecoil is a coil of wire within the hearing aid that picks up an induction signal (usually emitted from a telephone handset) and converts that back to sound. When you switch the hearing aid to the telecoil setting, the microphone turns off to eliminate competing noise and the telecoil looks for that induction signal.

Challenges with In-the-Ear (ITE) hearing aids

The smaller completely-in-the-canal hearing aids (CIC) and some ITE hearing aids provide adequate amplification and can be used with an existing headset without additional accommodations. These individuals may find the amplification available in the existing system adequate and can use the headsets without any feedback (or squealing).

Many individuals with ITE hearing aids find that the existing amplification within the system is not adequate and they struggle to hear clearly. They may also experience feedback when they place the headsets on. They may even remove their hearing aids to answer calls.

Challenges with Behind-the-Ear (BTE) hearing aids

The BTE style hearing aid cannot easily or effectively be used with existing headsets. There is a relatively new headset available that is designed for people with BTE hearing aids who have the telecoil option.

This headset uses an amplifier and a headset with special earpieces (called silhouettes) that are placed over the ear and rest directly next to the hearing aid. These earpieces create the induction signal that a telecoil needs to operate. The signal is very strong because the earpiece sits directly next to the hearing aid. The individual puts on the headset, places the earpieces next to his or her hearing aid and switches the hearing aids to telecoil.

Hearing Aids and Environmental Noises

Background noise in a call center can be very distracting to any person but can cause significant difficulty for a person wearing hearing aids. Hearing aids pick up all sounds, not just sound through the headset. It can be very beneficial to reduce the background noise.

Many employees perform better when they are situated at a station on the outside perimeter and away from file cabinets (sound reflects off of the metal cabinets), copy machines and off the main traffic areas. Full size fabric wall partitions also help reduce ambient room noise.

Another option that may be needed (or helpful in an interim period) is to allow only land-line calls to be answered. Land-line originated calls tend to have less background noise and a clearer signal. The incoming sig-

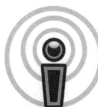

nal on cell phone calls are often very noisy, have static and background noise. This can be very difficult for any person, but the signal can be even more distorted when amplifying the sound for the person with hearing loss.

These no-cost, low cost environmental accommodations provide significant benefit. The individual with hearing loss may also benefit from more frequent breaks.

Amplifier Solutions

A Plantronics Vista M12 amplifier and headset are successful in providing amplification in many facilities. The amplifier plugs into the headset box at the computer (one brand is an ACS box). The headset itself plugs into the amplifier with a quick disconnect cable.

The Plantronics Encore headsets are effective for many people. The earpieces are replaced with slightly larger padded earpieces and provide a good seal around the ear.

There can be up to three different volume control switches to adjust. The computer may have a volume control setting, the headset box likely has a volume control and so does the M12 amplifier. The goal is to use the lowest volume settings possible to reduce potential distortion into the signal.

The recommended initial settings are as follows:

Computer – Set volume at 7 or 8

Headset box – Set volume at 3 (use this control SECOND to increase volume)

Amplifier – Set volume low (use this control FIRST to increase volume)

Headset Solutions

The style of hearing aid is crucial for lessening feedback and providing the most effective interface to the headset.

Some individuals will try and turn the hearing aid volume down slightly. But if the volume is turned too low, all benefit from the hearing aid programming is lost. The amplifiers just increase the volume while the hearing aid is programmed to increase those sounds the individual needs.

If feedback is still an issue after the volume settings on the computer, headset box, amplifier and hearing aid are adjusted, then a different set of hearing aids may be a solution.

Case Study

Ashley is a call center operator whose hearing has deteriorated and she struggles with phone calls. Management has noticed her numbers are dropping as calls seem to take longer. Ashley's performance is based on the number of completed calls and the call times.

Ashley does not yet have hearing aids and it may be awhile before she can afford them or before she is eligible for vocational rehabilitation services. Her desk is situated near a major traffic area that can be noisy at times.

The quietest area on the floor is in the back corner. Most of the cubicles have half or three-quarter high fabric walls. Ashley could move to the quietest area on the floor and perhaps have full paneled walls installed to help insulate against background noise.

She is currently using a single earpiece on the headphones. An amplifier like the Plantronics M12 amplifier can be installed at the headset box and a Plantronics Encore binaural headset can be used with the amplifier to provide volume increase. The binaural headsets provide sound to both ears while also helping to reduce background noise. These accommodations have been helpful for her moderate hearing loss.

Common Technical Accommodations

- Headset amplifier (like the Plantronics Vista M12)
- Binaural headphones (like Plantronics Encore)
- Hatis Director Headset with special cable for M12 amplifier
- Plantronics earpads for the headphones

ON THE JOB WITH HEARING LOSS
Hearing Loss Issues and Corrections Officers

The purpose of this report is to help you more fully identify potential communication barriers on the job. Each report focuses on a specific employment situation or topic and offers possible solutions to typical job functions. The combination of hearing instruments, assistive technology and communication strategies play a significant role in obtaining successful communication.

Corrections Officers

Communication Demands of Typical Job Functions

- Communicate with residents in loud environments
- Be aware of surroundings
- Hear on the telephone
- Hear on radios

Issues to Consider and Potential Accommodations

Communicating with residents is often difficult because most areas within a facility have concrete walls, reverberation and loud background noise. It is difficult to hear conversations and many individuals are uncomfortable speaking loudly to staff.

FM systems are helpful in these kinds of listening environments because the microphone can be placed closer to the person speaking while turning off the hearing aid microphone to help reduce the background noise while using the system. There are a few considerations with the technology that is available.

Officers may not want to use an assistive listening system that requires cords that could become a safety hazard. A neckloop can be used if the neckloop remains under clothing. The sound signal should be strong enough for the hearing aid telecoil. Another option is to use a wireless FM receiver that snaps onto a behind-the-ear hearing aid. The transmitter with microphone is handheld and can point towards the person speaking.

One other option is to use a device that is discreet and slips over one ear. It is called a Link-It and produces a signal for the hearing aid telecoil. It is a directional microphone and designed for one-on-one conversation in noisy environments. There is no handheld unit for this device. The Link-It looks like a pencil placed above the ear.

Be aware of surroundings. If the individual uses one of the options above with the hearing aid set on telecoil, they will not be able to hear co-workers because the hearing aid microphone turns off when the telecoil is turned on. If it is possible to have an M/T switch (microphone + telecoil) on the hearing aid, then he or she will be able to hear both environmental sounds plus the sound coming through the assistive listening system. Otherwise, they may set one hearing on telecoil while leaving the other one on microphone to pick up both environmental sounds and the sound through the FM system.

Hearing on 2-way radios can be challenging. Using a remote speaker that plugs into the radio and clips on the shoulder is effective in bringing the speaker closer to the ear. Sometimes administration may be reluctant to provide this because they feel everyone may want one, but it is a valid accommodation for someone with hearing loss.

Hearing conversations on the phone may easily be solved by trying an inline amplifier that fits between the handset and base of the telephone. This device provides both amplification and a stronger induction signal.

Case Study

Dwight is a corrections officer in a medium security facility. He has a moderate to severe hearing loss and is receiving new hearing aids. He must communicate with residents in the open area and monitor the cafeteria. He must communicate on the telephone and respond to his 2-way radio. Residents often speak softly and he finds it difficult to hear them in the noisy areas.

If Dwight gets BTE (behind-the-ear) hearing aids, he will be able to use a wireless FM system like the Microlink system that uses a handheld transmitter/microphone and a receiver that plugs directly into this hearing aid. The receiver can be set to FM only (for noisy backgrounds) or to FM + Hearing Aids so that he can hear everything. He likes the option of simply switching the receiver between the two settings.

If he gets ITE (in-the-ear) hearing aids with telecoils, he would have to use an FM system that uses a neckloop that he could wear under his shirt. He is not as comfortable with this option because he doesn't want a cord around his neck.

One other option that Dwight can try is an all-in-one small earpiece that slips over the ear and points forward. It is called a Link-It and will enhance sounds within 5-7 feet in front of

the person. It is designed to pick up sound with a directional microphone from someone standing nearby. Dwight would simply switch his ITE or BTE aid with telecoil on to the telecoil setting.

If Dwight's hearing loss were less severe, his audiologist may recommend completely in-the-canal (CIC) hearing aids. An FM system may not be necessary with CIC aids or it may be used with either an earhook or headphones.

Dwight will work with his audiologist to determine the best option based on his level of hearing loss.

Dwight also has difficulty understanding messages on the 2-way radio. Some officers already use shoulder speakers that are an accessory of the 2-way radio. Dwight will begin using this so that the sound is near his ear.

Common Technical Accommodations

- Hearing aids are the primary technology solution
- InfoLoop Portable Listening system for hearing aids with telecoils
- Inline phone amplifier
- FM system with a transmitter/microphone and a receiver with a listening option that gets the sound to the hearing aid or to the ear (Phonak Microlink or Lexis)
- Directional microphone (like the Link-It)
- Shoulder speaker accessory for 2 way radio

ON THE JOB WITH HEARING LOSS
Hearing Loss Issues and Factory Workers

The purpose of this report is to help you more fully identify potential communication barriers on the job. Each report focuses on a specific employment situation or topic and offers possible solutions to typical job functions. The combination of hearing instruments, assistive technology and communication strategies play a significant role in obtaining successful communication.

Factory Workers

People who work in factories must usually contend with loud machinery and background noise. Other challenges in the environment often include heat and humidity. These are 'hostile' environments for effective hearing aid use. Appropriate hearing protection is typically mandated.

Communication Demands of Typical Job Functions

- Be aware of safety warnings (such as fork lifts, etc).
- Hear co-workers or supervisor
- Participate in on-the-job training and staff meetings
- Understand clearly on the phone
- Hear intercom pages
- Communicate while wearing hearing protection

Issues to Consider

Being aware of safety warnings is of primary importance. There are no easy ways to send a signal from forklifts and other machinery to people with hearing loss. These individuals must rely on visual alerting such as the flashing light on the forklift. The installation of wide-angle mirrors at all intersections can provide additional safety for everyone, including the forklift driver. Marked paths on the floor for pedestrian traffic are also useful.

Using a tactile device may be helpful if the warehouse does not have loud background noise like factory machinery. The Tactaid device has microphones and it acts as a sound monitor. Vibrating discs are worn on the wrist. Training is necessary to learn the vibration pattern of specific sounds but may work as a secondary alerting device.

Emergency alerting for fire, etc. should also be visual. If this isn't possible, then the use of pagers may be helpful. If management uses text or numeric pagers, then one can be used by the person with hearing loss. A private paging system mentioned later is another option.

Ability to hear co-workers is also difficult. The efforts involved in meeting this challenge may be influenced by the communication demand. If speaking and listening is too difficult, pen and paper works well. If computers are located on the floor, the ability to bring up a blank screen so that you can type is also useful. See the discussion on hearing protection that follows.

On the job training is a vitally important step in advancing to higher paying positions. Start the training in a quiet room so the instructions can be read and issues discussed in this more advantageous setting. The individual with hearing loss is then better prepared to go out on the floor. Have all instructions typed and easily accessible on the floor for quick and easy reference.

If training videos are not captioned, the script should be transcribed and available for anyone who cannot hear the television. An assistive listening system can also be used for the television. All training courses should have good printed materials and all meetings should have written agendas.

Understanding clearly on the phone can be difficult. Most pay phones have volume control. An office phone in a quieter area with an inline telephone amplifier will also be helpful for anyone who has difficulty hearing in background noise. A pay-phone TTY can be installed that is vandal resistant or a TTY can be placed in an office area.

Staff meetings can be difficult for someone with a hearing loss. Obvious strategies include arriving early to get a position as close to the speaker as possible. If this isn't helpful, ask the speaker to arrange follow-up on key points after the meeting. If an FM system is used for other areas, then it can be used in this meeting as well. A portable amplifier/speaker has also been used to amplify the speaker's voice for everyone, specifically in the break room.

Hearing aids and hearing protection. There are many considerations:

- Conventional hearing protection typically improves speech intelligibility for normal hearing people. Hearing protection often degrades speech intelligibility for the person with hearing loss.

- There are two special hearing protection headsets with 23 NRR and 25 NRR that are successful. These are electronic headsets that provide enhanced communication without the need to remove the headset. These headsets have built-in microphones facing forward on each ear-cup. There is a volume control wheel that can be turned on to amplify the person speaking in front of the individual and then turned off when the conversation is over, thus restoring hearing protection.

- Find an audiologist in the area who will assist an employee with hearing loss. They will recommend the most workable solution based on the individual's level of hearing loss, the hearing aid currently in use, and the hearing protection that is needed.

- The use of an assistive listening system can provide a significant improvement in hearing the speaker's voice. The goal is to get a microphone as close to the speaker's lips as possible so that their voice is the primary sound. A one piece unit like the PockeTalker is feasible for occasional use. If a one piece unit is undesirable because of dirt, environment or wearing gloves, then use a two-piece unit such as an FM system.

- Heat and humidity can render hearing aids inoperable. The use of the headphones with speakers or an assistive listening system becomes even more important for protecting both hearing and the hearing aid.

- Use of a paging system with a vibrating receiver is sometimes highly effective. The base transmitter is placed at a common point. The person with hearing loss wears the vibrating receiver. To send a page, a person simply presses the button. This system operates up to 2 miles and may need an outside booster antenna depending on plant size and machinery.

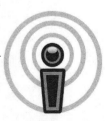

Case Study

John works at a station on an assembly line. He moves parts into the line area and moves finished product to another area. He must be able to hear the forklifts that drive by and must monitor several stations along a machine. He has a moderate to severe hearing loss and must hear if the machine breaks or jams. He must communicate with co-workers.

John cannot understand any announcements over the intercom. He wears hearing protection and removes it to hear someone speaking to him. He doesn't wear his hearing aids at work because of dirt and sweat. He has difficulty hearing during meetings in the break room and at lunch.

His manager has several concerns. John is often late to work because he oversleeps. He is also concerned for John's safety because of his inability to hear warning sounds or the sounds of the forklifts.

John purchased an alarm clock with a vibrating disc that slips under his mattress. Now he no longer depends on the audible alarm.

He began using an electronic hearing protection headset with microphones on the ear cups that face forward. He can turn on the microphones with a control knob and the sound in front of him is amplified through the speakers built into the headset. The headset then returns to full hearing protection when he turns it off. People need to be somewhat close to him, but he doesn't need to remove the headset now.

If John has in-the-ear hearing aids, his audiologist may agree that he can safely keep his hearing aids in while using the hearing protection headset. He uses a system that removes moisture from the hearing aid overnight.

Common Technical Accommodations

- Inline phone amplifier
- TTY
- Personal amplifier (like PockeTalker) or FM system
  - Private Page personal paging system
  - Bilsom hearing protection headset

- Williams Sound Hearing Protection headset to use with PockeTalker or FM system
- Portable PA system
- Vibrating alarm clock
- Wide angle mirrors at intersections
- Dry and Store hearing aid conditioner

ON THE JOB WITH HEARING LOSS
Hearing Loss Issues and Food Service Workers

The purpose of this report is to help you more fully identify potential communication barriers on the job. Each report focuses on a specific employment situation or topic and offers possible solutions to typical job functions. The combination of hearing instruments, assistive technology and communication strategies play a significant role in obtaining successful communication.

Food Service Workers

There are three types of food service positions that are difficult: Working behind the counter with equipment, working behind the counter with customers and working out on the floor with customers. Each presents different challenges. There are unique issues and solutions for each position.

Communication Demands of Typical Job Functions
- Understand customers while out on the floor
- Hear customers and co-workers from behind a counter
- Hear oven timers, buzzers, etc

Issues to Consider

Knowing what customers are saying is vitally important. It is difficult to hear someone place an order or make a request when the restaurant is crowded and there is competing background noise.

If hearing instruments alone aren't helpful in this situation, the use of a personal listening system like a PockeTalker may be helpful. The unit has a microphone and can be placed in a pocket or on the waistband. Simply place the microphone closer to the person speaking when it is difficult to hear someone. The speaker's voice will be amplified more than the background noise. The listening option delivers the sound to the ear or the hearing aid.

Helpful communication strategies. It can be helpful to be open about your hearing loss when asking someone to repeat. Practice saying "I have a hearing loss and it helps if you speak a bit louder (or slower, etc)." Also verify and confirm what you *did* hear so that the customer does not need to repeat everything. Many people say using these strategies provides added benefit because their customers feel they really care and are trying harder to meet their needs. Chapter 7 provides excellent guidelines that can improve the communication process.

Understanding the customer from behind a counter also presents a challenge. There is usually background noise to deal with as well. Hearing instruments with directional microphones may be helpful. The use of an assistive listening system can also be helpful. A well-placed microphone on a gooseneck stand facing the customer will deliver a clear sound signal to the ear or hearing aids. The FM system with separate microphone and receiver units allows freedom of movement. Hearing instruments with telecoils can often provide additional benefit in controlling background noise.

Hearing audible alarms is the most difficult situation to accommodate. There are some types of equipment that use colored lights or flashing lights for notification in addition to audible alarms. This equipment is easier to work with. Sometimes an engineer can modify an audible alarm to activate a light.

Another option is to use a paging system for close range. The person with hearing loss wears a vibrating receiver. A paging unit can be mounted or worn by a co-worker. The co-worker presses the paging button and the receiver vibrates to signal the employee. This system can indicate 4 different 'instructions' by using 4 separate paging buttons. These 4 different icons will light on the vibrating receiver to indicate the instruction. This system is also useful for employees who don't have hearing loss but who require prompting from a manager or co-worker.

Hearing instruments can provide tremendous benefit. Be sure the hearing health care professional understands the work environment. There are hearing instruments that can provide significant benefit, including programmable hearing instruments and directional microphones. The hearing healthcare professional can recommend the most appropriate and useful technology based on the individual's level of hearing loss.

Case Study

Jane has a moderate to severe hearing loss and works in a school cafeteria. She wears hearing aids but while she works in the kitchen during food preparation, she cannot hear co-workers at a distance because of exhaust fans. She doesn't hear the timers and co-workers yell to get her attention. Jane also works the cash register and must be able to hear children when they speak with her or give her their lunch code.

Jane received new hearing aids while working with the department of vocational rehabilitation. Her new hearing aids have directional microphones that help her hear at the cash register. She made several trips back to the audiologist to adjust the hearing aids to give her optimum performance while working in the kitchen with the background noise. Her co-workers can call out her name to get her attention now.

Another option that works for a food service worker named Mary is the use of an FM system. One co-worker wears the FM transmitter with lapel microphone and Mary wears the FM receiver and an earhook that covers one ear. The earhook is a small ear speaker that hangs over one ear like half of a headphone. Mary is able to use this option without the hearing aid squealing.

The co-worker's voice is amplified over the background noise and Mary is able to hear clearly. The FM system lapel microphone is attached to a gooseneck stand next to the cash register. When Mary works the register, she attaches the FM transmitter to it and is better able to hear customers as they come through the hospital cafeteria line.

Common Technical Accommodations

- Personal pagers and receivers from Silent Call Corporation

- FM system with a transmitter/microphone and a receiver with a listening option that gets the sound to the hearing aid or to the ear

- Portable InfoLoop induction listening system

- Personal amplifier (like PockeTalker)

ON THE JOB WITH HEARING LOSS
Hearing Loss Issues and Home Health Care Personnel

The purpose of this report is to help you more fully identify potential communication barriers on the job. Each report focuses on a specific employment situation or topic and offers possible solutions to typical job functions. The combination of hearing instruments, assistive technology and communication strategies play a significant role in obtaining successful communication.

Home Health Care Personnel

The home health care profession is a growing field. Home health aides take on a variety of tasks that require good communication skills because of the number of people with whom they come in contact. It is essential that they hear clearly.

Communication Demands of Typical Job Functions

- Hear clients in one-on-one situations

- Hear on a telephone or cell phone

- Use a stethoscope

Issues to Consider

Personal Care or Companionship/Homemaking Services
Home care workers must hear their client during one-on-one conversations and from another room if necessary. Hearing aids are the first choice accommodation. Additional accommodations may include a personal listening system to enhance one-on-one conversations or a phone amplifier so that any telephone is accessible.

Home care workers may use a cell phone for their communications and the ability to hear clearly on the cell phone is important. If cell phone use is a challenge, then refer to Chapter 4 – Dealing with Telephones to understand the options available. The options vary depending on the level of hearing loss, type of hearing aids used and model of cell phone.

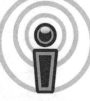

Skilled nursing care

Home health care workers such as nurses and speech or occupational thera-pists have the same one-on-one listening challenges. Nurses may also need to use a stethoscope. Amplified stethoscopes are available for people with or without hearing aids. See the report, "Hearing Loss Issues and Medical Pro-fessionals" for more detailed information on the stethoscope issue.

Case Study

Marie is 46 years old and has a moderate hearing loss. She has thought about purchasing hearing aids, but the cost is prohibitive at this time.

Marie feels that there are only a few areas that are difficult because of her hearing loss. When she talks with a client, she makes sure that the TV vol-ume is turned down or turned off to reduce distracting background noise. She usually sits facing the client so that she can speech-read, even though she doesn't know that is what it is called.

Marie may not realize that it is very difficult for her clients to get her at-tention if she walks into another room. Marie also works as a personal aide when necessary. The most difficult part of this job is that she cannot hear if the client calls out to her from the bedroom or other room. She needs to be alerted when someone calls out to her.

Marie now uses a personal amplifier when talking with clients and notices a significant improvement in speech understanding. She does not have to ask the client to repeat herself. She can go from room to room and hear when her name is called if she uses an FM system instead of a personal amplifier. She also carries a personal paging system so that her client sim-ply presses a button and a receiver that Marie wears vibrates to alert her.

Marie also found a phone amplifier that she can simply attach to a home phone if she needs to make a phone call. However, she prefers to use her new cell phone that has clear and loud sound.

Common Technical Accommodations

- Personal amplifier (like the PockeTalker)
  - Inline phone amplifier
  - Personal paging system (like Silent Call)

ON THE JOB WITH HEARING LOSS
Hearing Loss Issues and Inside Services and Salespersons

The purpose of this report is to help you more fully identify potential communication barriers on the job. Each report focuses on a specific employment situation or topic and offers possible solutions to typical job functions. The combination of hearing instruments, assistive technology and communication strategies play a significant role in obtaining successful communication.

Inside Services and Salespersons (insurance, real estate, accounting/bookkeeping)

Several occupations that include sales and service have similar communication demands: Hear customers in an office setting and outdoors, use the telephone and participate in continuing education. Successful sales reps rely on good communication skills to retain clients. These individuals are often self-employed.

Communication Demands of Typical Job Functions

- Hear the phone ring
- Hear conversations on the phone
- Hear customers in the office setting
- Participate in continuing education

Issues to Consider

Hearing the phone ring can be a challenge in an open office environment. The person with hearing loss may hear a phone ringing, but not be able to tell whose phone is ringing when away from their desk. An adjustable phone ringer can share the phone jack at the wall. The warble of the ring can be changed to more easily identify the ring. A phone signaler and vibrating personal receiver is also an option and has a 100 foot range.

Hearing clearly on the phone is essential. Individuals in these professions must clearly understand details. Misunderstandings can be costly. An inline phone amplifier can be used on almost any office phone. If the phone line is analog (not digital), then a specialty amplified phone can be used.
Refer to Chapter 4 – Telephones for more information.

The ability to hear in one-on-one listening situations is critical. Almost all communication with clients is either on the telephone or in an office setting. Hearing aids are the most useful accommodation but a personal amplifier can also enhance hearing. Place a conference microphone or an FM system transmitter's lapel microphone on the desk (or have the client wear the lapel microphone.)

Professional development is required to maintain licensing. Favorable seating near the front of the room is helpful. Using an assistive listening system is also helpful because the system helps overcome distance from the speaker and room reverberation. Request an assistive listening system at the time of registration so that the conference planner can secure accommodations.

Case Study

Gene is a realtor. He relies on the telephone to set appointments and contact clients. Lately, he has experienced several incidents lately that rattled him. Several clients called while waiting for him to arrive at a house. Gene wrote down a different time and had to hustle to meet them.

Gene does not connect these misunderstandings to a hearing loss because he feels sure that he hears fine in one-on-one conversations. However, his wife is not surprised when he tells her about these incidents. She often tells him he only hears when he wants to. Many arguments have ensued because of misunderstandings. She says, "I told you about that." He says, "No, you didn't."

Gene has a mild to moderate hearing loss. He understands clearly when speaking one-on-one with customers or family. He does not realize he is missing conversations when his wife speaks to him from the kitchen while he is watching TV or when the dishwasher is running. These background noises interfere with his ability to hear. Telephone amplifiers easily improve the issues with telephone conversations.

Common Technical Accommodations

- Inline phone amplifier

- Adjustable phone ringer

- Telephone transmitter and personal vibrating receiver

- Cell phone interface

- FM system with a transmitter/microphone and a receiver with a listening option that gets the sound to the hearing aid or to the ear

- Personal amplifier (like PockeTalker) with conference microphone

ON THE JOB WITH HEARING LOSS
Hearing Loss Issues and Maintenance Personnel

The purpose of this report is to help you more fully identify potential communication barriers on the job. Each report focuses on a specific employment situation or topic and offers possible solutions to typical job functions. The combination of hearing instruments, assistive technology and communication strategies play a significant role in obtaining successful communication.

Maintenance, Janitorial and Housekeeping positions

Maintenance personnel face a variety of communication challenges. They usually work throughout a facility, communicate on a 2 way radio, hear building alarms and communicate one-on-one. Hearing aids generally provide significant improvement, but obstacles exist for people with more severe hearing loss.

Communication Demands of Typical Job Functions

- Hear and respond to a 2-way radio
- Hear building alarms and overhead pages
- Converse with co-workers one-on-one

Issues to Consider

People with hearing loss find 2-way radios difficult to understand. If they cannot tell that the message is for them, use a simple code or phrase. Repeat the phrase twice. For example; instead of saying, "John, please come to the front office", the initial phrase "John, 1, 2, 3, or John Simpson" is repeated. John can then identify the message is for him.

Building alarms and overhead pages can cause similar problems. The same process used for 2-way radios are used for overhead pages. Another option for notification is to use a vibrating pager. A vibrating pager system, similar to the ones in restaurants, will cause a pager to vibrate when a transmitted code is sent. These systems have up to a 2-mile range. If additional distance is needed, purchase an outside or mountable antenna for extended range. The transmitting base unit is often placed in a receptionist office where there is always coverage. Anyone who needs to page the individual can call the office and the receptionist can simply press the transmit button. A 0-9 single digit display is pre-coded so that everyone knows what the code means.

The paging system can also be used to notify the individual with hearing loss who is using a 2-way radio that the call is for him. This is especially useful if there is loud background noise that will interfere with that individual's ability to hear on the radio or phone.

Communicating with co-workers is important. Hearing aids alone may be the best technology available for one-on-one or close communications. When background noise interferes with clear understanding, a personal amplifier is helpful.

Case Study

Charlie is a general maintenance worker in a nursing home. He uses his 2-way radio with the receptionist and one other co-worker. He is usually able to understand the radio in most of the areas of the facility. There are a few areas, however, that are difficult for him because of background noise. Sometimes he is not sure if the message is for him or his co-worker.

Charlie found that the strategy of saying his first and last name and pausing before continuing the message helps him identify the call is for him. He will try to find a quiet area to talk.

Kat on the other hand performs janitorial duties and must respond to the 2-way radio. She has a severe hearing loss and has difficulty understanding the radio. There are several co-workers with the 2-way radios and many of the calls across the radio are not for Kat. Kat tried the messaging strategy but so many people used the radio and they would often forget.

The company installed a paging system in the front office. People who need to contact Kat call the front office. The receptionist in turn transmits a code to Kat. Code 1 indicates a call is coming in to Kat, Code 9 is a building alarm alert so that Kat can take appropriate action.

Kat also used a remote shoulder speaker for the radio so that the speaker was closer to her ear.

Kat could use the paging system for notification and then a phone amplifier so that she could use any telephone in-house without using a 2-way radio.

Common Technical Accommodations

- Private Page paging system with vibrating receiver

- Inline phone amplifier

- Shoulder speaker radio accessory

- Personal amplifier (like PockeTalker) for one-on-one communications

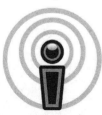

ON THE JOB WITH HEARING LOSS
Hearing Loss Issues and Managers

The purpose of this report is to help you more fully identify potential communication barriers on the job. Each report focuses on a specific employment situation or topic and offers possible solutions to typical job functions. The combination of hearing instruments, assistive technology and communication strategies play a significant role in obtaining successful communication.

Managers

Individuals in management positions often face similar difficult situations. Of course, specific job duties may vary. The individual's first step should be to see a hearing healthcare professional if he or she does not already have hearing aids. Hearing instruments make a tremendous difference in most areas of performance.

Communication Demands of Typical Job Functions

- Lead meetings and participate in meetings
- Communicate clearly on the telephone
- Communicate with staff in casual settings and in social situations
- Travel independently
- Attend workshops and conferences

Issues to Consider

Ability to lead or participate in meetings. One-on-one meetings with staff are a breeze and small meetings may be easy to navigate. Attendance at a larger meeting or leading a meeting can be more difficult. Managers often feel they appear ineffective or incapable when they continually ask people to repeat or if they respond inappropriately to a question or line of conversation. Chapter 6 addresses meeting situations and offers excellent strategies for more effective meetings.

Understanding clearly on the phone can be difficult. An inline telephone amplifier is the most common accommodation employers provide. If the amplifier provided is not clear or loud enough, then quality in-line amplifiers are available through assistive device (or ALD) vendors.

Business travel is often stressful. The need to understand overhead pages, hear taxi drivers, use pay phones and wake up in the morning are communication issues all travelers face. Telling the taxi driver you are hard of hearing and asking them to speak a little louder from the front seat may be helpful. Bringing a strap-on phone amplifier that fits on any telephone gives you access to any phone.

There are assistive devices that are particularly suited to travel. A vibrating alarm clock and a door knock signaler are accommodations that must be provided by the hotel with prior notification under the Americans with Disabilities Act.

Attendance at conferences is often required and communication is always challenging. There are individual sessions with moderate sized groups and one main speaker. There are round table discussions. During the luncheon, the need to hear the main speaker or panel of speakers as well as others at the table is necessary.

The combination of appropriate hearing instruments and the ability to use an FM system allows fuller participation and a richer experience. By placing the FM system microphone close to the desired sound source at the front of the room, the speech signal is amplified. The sound is transmitted to the receiver and this increase in the speech signal overcomes background noise and distance from the speaker.

Reluctance to Use of Hearing Aids and Denial of the Hearing Loss

Managers often feel that wearing hearing aids make them appear old, unable to do their jobs, or less intelligent. Counseling is often helpful and necessary to help people accept their hearing loss and take steps to improve their ability to communicate.

You cannot hide hearing loss and negative repercussions occur when the issue is not addressed. Recognizing the hearing loss and taking positive steps to improve communication puts you in control of the process. Hearing aids, assistive technology and communication strategies (along with a little patience and humor) are tools that help you become your own problem solver.

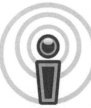

Case Study

John is 57 years old and is reluctantly pursuing hearing aids and assistive technology after his supervisor suggested he work with the vocational rehabilitation agency. John thinks his hearing isn't really that bad. He doesn't see his hearing loss as a problem and fears hearing aids will undermine his reputation.

John attends many meetings in various offices with groups from 6 to 60 people. He often walks with customers through the warehouse and feels he manages well. He is able to use the telephone with volume control in his office.

John's supervisor listed some areas of concern. He heard co-workers complain that John didn't listen to them and often seemed uninterested in their conversations. John seemed reluctant to participate during some of the meetings. It seemed that his performance was slipping. John and his supervisor reviewed the information and that is why they sought help from a vocational rehabilitation counselor.

John didn't purposely hide his loss and honestly felt he was managing well. He didn't realize that he walked past people who had called out his name or didn't respond to jokes or stories when others were socializing. It was simply because he didn't hear them or they didn't get his attention first before speaking.

John is learning how his hearing loss was affecting his job and that he was NOT managing the hearing loss as well as he thought. While he felt that hearing aids would alert everyone that he had a hearing loss, he soon realized that everyone already knew he did.

John has a moderate hearing loss and his audiologist recommend hearing aids. They are effective in almost every listening situation except in larger meetings. John finds that simple communication rules help as well. He often reminds people to get his attention before talking to him. He is now using meeting rules.

John can hear people next to him during meetings but has trouble hearing people from the far end of the table. An FM system is used for this situation with a conference microphone placed at the other end of the table. John hears more clearly because of the microphone placement and participates more fully.

John is successful in using hearing aids, communication strategies and an FM system to meet most of his communication needs. If his hearing loss had been more severe, John would use the FM system more often.

Common Technical Accommodations

- FM system with a transmitter/microphone and a receiver with a listening option that gets the sound to the hearing aid or to the ear and a conference microphone

- Inline phone amplifier or strap-on amplifier

- Alerting system for travel for alarm clock, door knock, telephone

- Vibrating alarm clock

ON THE JOB WITH HEARING LOSS
Hearing Loss Issues and Medical Personnel

The purpose of this report is to help you more fully identify potential communication barriers on the job. Each report focuses on a specific employment situation or topic and offers possible solutions to typical job functions. The combination of hearing instruments, assistive technology and communication strategies play a significant role in obtaining successful communication.

Medical Personnel

Medical personnel who must use a stethoscope regularly report difficulty in finding a stethoscope that can work when hearing aids are in. Almost every hearing aid wearer dislikes removing his or her hearing aids each time they use the stethoscope. Other difficulties frequently reported include hearing soft-spoken or weak patients, hearing overhead pages and distinguishing where alarm sounds are originating. Telephone use can also be a problem, especially in a noisy station.

Communication Demands of Typical Job Functions

- Use a stethoscope
- Understand clearly on the phone (especially doctor's orders)
- Hear weak or soft-spoken patients
- Respond to alarm sounds from medical equipment
- Respond to overhead pages

Issues to Consider

Stethoscope usage is the number one priority by nursing personnel at all levels. A primary goal for medical professionals is the ability to keep the hearing aids in while using the stethoscope. Most professionals do not want to remove their hearing aids because of sanitation reasons and the increased risk of losing the aids. If a medical professional does not wear hearing instruments, an amplified stethoscope may be all that is needed.

There are several amplified stethoscopes on the market. A few will interface with hearing aids and allow the hearing aids to remain in the ear.

This interface also allows someone with a significant hearing loss the ability to use the stethoscope because it uses the full power of the hearing aid.

If hearing instruments are purchased at the time the stethoscope is addressed, then effective interfaces may be possible with the hearing aid earmold or options. The report **"How to Cope with Scopes"** shares up-to-date information on stethoscope options and hearing aid options. Share this report with the hearing healthcare professional.

Understanding clearly on the phone is critical when speaking with a doctor. Nurses' stations can be noisy and hearing on the phone more difficult. Hearing aids may cause feedback or squealing. First, work with the hearing aid professional to address the feedback issues or to provide telecoil training if the hearing aids have telecoils. Using a telephone amplifier increases the volume and the signal strength and provides an effective accommodation.

Hearing weak or soft-spoken patients can be a challenge. Hearing instruments will be most helpful in this situation as well as in hearing in general. Soft-spoken individuals are hard to understand and the use of a personal amplifier allows a medical professional to place the microphone closer to the patient's mouth to get the best signal possible and amplify soft sounds.

Responding to equipment alarms is also difficult. There are no assistive devices that can really help this situation. Most all alarms are a high frequency pitch. Hearing instruments may help if the hard of hearing person doesn't already wear them. The only recourse is to continue to walk the hall to monitor and identify the location of the sound.

Hearing overhead pages can be difficult. Many medical personnel work in facilities with long hallways that are a distance form the nurse's station. A paging system is often helpful in this situation to communicate with the individual on the floor. A base station sits at the nurse's station. The nurse on the floor wears a vibrating receiver. When a code is pressed into the transmitter, the receiver vibrates and the code is displayed. This is an effective, inexpensive communication device that eliminates the reliance of speech understanding over a paging/intercom system.

Concerns in the 'real' world. Many nurses try to hide their hearing loss which increases the stress. They have legitimate concerns about their job security. With the appropriate use of technology and hearing aids, it is possible to continue full nursing duties. Amplified stethoscopes, amplified telephones, paging systems and assistive listening systems are reasonable job accommodations.

The Association of Medical Professionals with Hearing Losses is an online community providing information, promoting advocacy and mentorship and encouraging communication among individuals with hearing loss working in the health care fields. Access more information at www.amphl.org.

Case Study

Jan is an RN who has had an increasingly difficult time performing her job duties as her hearing loss progressed to a severe loss. She cannot hear the IV pump or the call buttons and struggles to hear on the phone, especially doctors with heavy accents. The background noise where the phone is located can sometimes be very loud.

Jan also has a difficult time when she comes on shift for the report meeting. She can hear some of the others in the room, but there are a few people who have soft voices. She is also concerned that she might not be hearing everything she needs to with the stethoscope.

There have been instances where experienced RNs have retired early because they couldn't deal with the stress of not hearing well and did not know of any technology to help them. Jan is considering early retirement.

Jan is fortunate because her supervisor and co-workers are supportive of her and helped her find potential accommodations. She received hearing aids that greatly improved much of the difficulties she was having.

She still cannot hear the IV pumps, or cannot localize the sounds. She uses a phone amplifier and communication strategies such as clarifying or verifying the information from the doctors. She uses an FM system in the meetings and places a conference microphone at the far end of the table to hear those people better.

Jan found an amplified stethoscope that allowed her to keep her hearing aids in while using the scope. She doesn't have to worry about losing the hearing aids or introducing them to un-sterile conditions. The stethoscope uses headphones that allow her to set the headphones over her ear with her hearing aids in. Jan also learned of the Association of Medical Professionals with Hearing Losses and visits their website and forum regularly for support and advice from other nurses with hearing loss.

Common Technical Accommodations

- Amplified stethoscope with headphones in-the-ear hearing aids or different listening options behind-the-ear hearing aids or cochlear implant

- Inline phone amplifier

- FM system with a transmitter/microphone and a receiver with environmental microphone and a listening option that gets the sound to the hearing aid or to the ear

- Private Page paging system or in-facility paging system

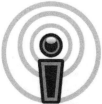

ON THE JOB WITH HEARING LOSS
Hearing Loss Issues and Office Personnel

The purpose of this report is to help you more fully identify potential communication barriers on the job. Each report focuses on a specific employment situation or topic and offers possible solutions to typical job functions. The combination of hearing instruments, assistive technology and communication strategies play a significant role in obtaining successful communication.

Office Personnel

Administrative assistants, clerks and almost anyone in an office environment face similar communication difficulties. The top complaint from most office workers is the inability to use the phone effectively. Noisy environments and meetings round out the top 3 areas that cause stress and affect job performance.

Communication Demands of Typical Job Functions

- Hear conversations on the phone
- Know when the phone rings
- Hear customers/coworkers during regular office conversations
- Hear in meetings, especially when asked to take notes

Issues to Consider

Telephone usage is the number one priority and complaint by many office workers. Telephone amplifiers are the number one requested accommodation to employers. Often an employee finds that a replacement handset does not provide enough improvement. There are two universal in-line amplifiers that work with most office phones. They give from 20-40 dB volume gain and provide significant improvement to most office phones.

If an individual wears hearing aids and the feedback or squealing prevents them from using the phone effectively, they should speak with their hearing healthcare provider. Also, foam telephone earpads may be effective in reducing the feedback.

If a person has tried to use the phone with their hearing aid telecoil and it just doesn't seem strong enough, they should try an inline amplifier. These units not only increase the sound, but they also boost the signal that the telecoil needs to perform better.

It is important to know when the phone is ringing. It is often difficult to hear or distinguish which telephone is ringing in an open office environment. A visual signaler can flash a lamp for alerting if the phone line is an analog line. An adjustable tone ringer is another option to help distinguish one phone from another one.

Digital phone lines offer fewer options. Signalers are often not sensitive enough to pick up the weaker signals from digital lines. Sound monitors don't always work well for office telephones because the sound coming from the newer electronic telephones is not strong enough to trigger the signaler.

One option is to change the phone port to analog (something the phone company handles) so that signalers will work. Another option is to try a sound monitor like the baby cry signaler to pick up the audible ring of the phone if you are in a quiet office. The sound signaler can alert you by either flashing a lamp plugged into a remote receiver or vibrating a personal, belt-worn receiver.

Participating in office conversations can be a real struggle. Some people find themselves shying away from groups because they are afraid of being embarrassed by answering incorrectly or altogether missing the point.

One factor in job performance is how well an employee relates and works with their coworkers. Hearing instruments or a personal amplifier can provide significant improvement in how well an individual can hear others.

Meetings can be difficult. Chapter 6 addresses meeting situations and offers excellent strategies for more effective meetings. Assistive listening systems are designed specifically to improve the speech signal and reduce background noise by placing the microphone close to the desired sound source.

Case Study

Charlotte works as a manager's assistant in an open office setting. She answers both her phone and her manager's phone. Conversations are informal among co-workers and Charlotte needs to hear these conversations. She meets with her manager and can hear in this one-on-one situation.

Charlotte has trouble noticing conversations that start informally. She often misses the first part of any conversation. She also struggles to hear on the phone, especially if people are talking in the background.

Charlotte finds a telephone amplifier that fits in between the handset and base of her phone provides good amplification. She reminds her co-workers to get her attention before they start talking. She reminds them "She needs to see them to hear them."

Charlotte has a moderate hearing loss and hearing aids provide significant improvement. If she were in an office that had more background noise, desk rearrangement or cubicle walls would be recommended to reduce the noise.

Common Technical Accommodations

- Inline phone amplifier

- Personal amplifier (like PockeTalker)

- FM system with a transmitter/microphone and a receiver with a listening option that gets the sound to the hearing aid or to the ear

- Adjustable phone ring tone signaler

ON THE JOB WITH HEARING LOSS
Hearing Loss Issues and Outdoor Workers

The purpose of this report is to help you more fully identify potential communication barriers on the job. Each report focuses on a specific employment situation or topic and offers possible solutions to typical job functions. The combination of hearing instruments, assistive technology and communication strategies play a significant role in obtaining successful communication.

Outdoor Workers (construction worker, equipment operator, farmer)

Individuals who work outdoors face similar communication challenges. Weather, background noise and distance from the person speaking are usually the biggest challenges. Technology must be resistant to heat, humidity and handling.

Communication Demands of Typical Job Functions

- Hear instructions or conversation from co-workers

- Hear the 2 way radio or cell phone

- Hear conversations when hearing protection or hard hats are necessary

Issues to Consider

Hearing aids are the most important technology for hearing instructions or conversations of co-workers and for monitoring equipment sounds. Hearing aids do not perform as well in heat and humidity and this can be a factor in which style of hearing aid is recommended by the hearing professional. The use of hearing aid covers and a good dehumidifier will be critical to successful performance of the hearing aids.

Using 2 way radios or cell phones can become more difficult if someone is trying to interface a hearing aid to the phone or radio. Many popular radios offer a shoulder speaker as an output from the radio. This shoulder speaker brings the sound closer to the ear and may even have an output jack for a direct cable or silhouette earpiece. Cell phone use is more convenient for a hearing aid user if either a neckloop is used to create a sound signal for hearing aid telecoils or if wireless Bluetooth technology is used.

Hearing protection headsets can be mounted onto hard hats or worn in the over-the-head style. Electronic headsets have forward facing microphones and a control to turn on the microphones. The headphones have ear speakers that will allow sound to enter the headset. The microphones can then be turned off to resume full hearing protection.

An FM system may also be used with the hearing protection headset if necessary. It will not provide 2 way communications, but can be used for notification and basic instruction. This electronic system should have a good warranty and able to withstand use.

Communicating with a person with severe to profound hearing loss is more challenging when working outdoors. Persons with hearing loss may not benefit from radio or cell phone communication. They must rely on the speaker getting their attention first so that they may speech read or read instructions. Some sign language knowledge among co-workers can help in basic communication if the employee uses ASL.

A paging system is helpful to get the attention of the employee with hearing loss. Use radios and cell phone with vibration. There are no paging devices for one-on-one paging with more than a 100-foot transmission range.

Case Study

Mitchell works mainly outdoors in construction. He often works on equipment used for roadside construction. Background noise from traffic and the machinery running limits his ability to hear and understand co-workers. He must wear hearing protection.

Mitchell has a severe hearing loss. Electronic hearing protection headsets offer the ability to mask out low or high frequency sounds while improving speech understanding. The forward facing microphones on the earcups are helpful in understanding co-workers when they come close.

Mitchell does not wear his hearing aids on the job because of sweat and weather conditions. He still needs help understanding speech. Since most of his communication is close or one-on-one, he uses a personal amplifier plugged into the hearing protection headset. This helps place the microphone closer to the person speaking.

Mitchell and his co-workers have devised hand signals to aid in communication. He also wears a 2-way radio set on vibration mode. If others need to get his attention, they call him to get his attention. No other technology at this time works well for him.

Common Technical Accommodations

- 2 way radio or cell phone set on vibration.
- Hands free headset or interface to hearing aids from the radio or cell phone.
- Personal amplifier (like PockeTalker)
- Electronic hearing protection headset with communication ability.

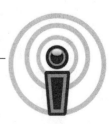

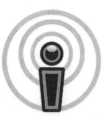

ON THE JOB WITH HEARING LOSS
Hearing Loss Issues and Pastors

The purpose of this report is to help you more fully identify potential communication barriers on the job. Each report focuses on a specific employment situation or topic and offers possible solutions to typical job functions. The combination of hearing instruments, assistive technology and communication strategies play a significant role in obtaining successful communication.

Pastors

Pastors and nurses with hearing loss share some common difficulties. Most counseling situations occur in one-on-one settings which are usually the easiest to handle. However, pastors often communicate with people who may not speak loudly or clearly because of emotional situations or because of illness.

Communication Demands of Typical Job Functions

- Counsel congregation members

- Lead services

- Participate in meetings

- Attend conferences or other functions that usually include a large group of people

- Use the telephone at work and in public facilities

- Know when the phone or doorbell rings when working alone in the office

Issues to Consider

Counseling situations are difficult. Hearing instruments may provide adequate benefit, but often an assistive listening system is very appropriate. An FM system works well by asking the speaker to clip the microphone to his or her lapel so that the receiver can amplify the sound. This is the most useful method of using the FM system. If it isn't feasible to ask someone to clip on the microphone, arrange the office so that the microphone can be clipped to an object on the desk as close to the individual as possible.

During services, pastors can enjoy the same benefits that members of the congregation enjoy from an assistive listening system. An FM system that connects to the existing PA system can transmit the sound signal to all receivers in the church. The pastor doesn't need the system to listen to his own sermon, but to hear the music and others who speak through the microphones.

Meetings are difficult, especially with large groups of individuals. Learn more about dealing with meetings from Chapter 6. The ability to control the environment and use effective communication strategies and an assistive listening system can improve communication access.

Large groups of people and background noise are a hostile combination for someone with hearing loss. Hearing instruments with directional microphones and assistive listening systems are helpful in these situations. Be sure to share this particular situation with your hearing health care provider. They may be able to solve many of these situations with programmable aids or aids with directional microphones. They may recommend hearing aids with telecoils or direct audio input so that the speech signal from an FM system is heard at the same time environmental sounds are picked up from the hearing aid.

Telephone access is important. Most church office phones have analog phone lines. A simple in-line amplifier may provide significant improvement by attaching it between the handset and the base of the phone. The telephone is then accessible.

Pastors often travel and need to use any available telephone. Most public pay phones have volume control buttons on them. A portable strap-on amplifier will make any phone more accessible. An amplified neckloop can be used with cellular phones if the hearing aid has telecoils.

When a pastor is alone in the office, it is important that he know when someone is at the door or when the phone is ringing. A fairly simple door alerting system allows the office door to be locked. When visitors push the doorbell button, a lamp attached to the signaler will flash. Phone calls will trigger the signaler to flash as well. There is a personal belt-worn receiver that will vibrate when either signal occurs. This only works up to 80 feet from the base system but may be a useful option.

FM Systems In Church:

How many members of the church congregation have hearing difficulties? How many older members have stopped coming to church because they can't hear or participate? Making church services accessible helps include everyone. Don't forget church functions and group studies. You can use the same FM system in other areas of the church with a few additional components.

Case Study

Pastor Ron has a moderate-to-severe hearing loss. He has just received hearing aids that have a telecoil and directional microphones. With hearing aids, he is able to hear almost everyone he meets in personal counsel because his office is quiet. He only has difficulty if the person has a weak voice or there is background noise around him.

The pastor leads the church service and delivers sermons. He must hear anyone else who is using the lectern as well as hear the choir. Often times he must hear members who ask him to pray for them. He cannot hear people beyond the front two rows. It is important to him that he hears the prayer requests. Hearing aids alone won't help in this situation, but an FM system will.

The FM system works like this: Pastor Ron enlists the help of someone else in the church to repeat any prayer requests, etc. into a microphone/transmitter. Pastor Ron is wearing the receiver and a neckloop. He switches one hearing aid to telecoil. The request is repeated into the microphone and he is able to hear it through the hearing aid's telecoil.

Pastor Ron must also attend many functions with large groups of people. This is the absolute hardest listening situation for him because of the background noise and people speaking to him from any side. Hearing aids with directional microphones will likely provide the most help.

If this doesn't help and he is struggling, an FM system can work. Pastor Ron wears a receiver and a neckloop to listen through his telecoils, but the receiver also has a microphone on it so that it can amplify sounds close to him. This is more cumbersome, but it eases some of the stress of listening in an 'unfriendly' listening environment.

The door to the church office is locked when Ron is the only person there. He will be using a special doorbell that will cause a signaler inside the office to flash to alert him that someone is at the door. There is also a phone signaler sharing a phone jack that will cause a signaler inside the office to flash as well. These signalers work up to 100 feet away. He may prefer a vibrating receiver to notify him of these sounds instead of a flashing lamp.

Common Technical Accommodations

- Alertmaster doorbell/phone signaler with wireless doorbell.

- Alertmaster vibrating receiver that is worn like a pager for phone/door alerting.

- Inline phone amplifier.

- Hearing Helper FM System with transmitter/microphone and receiver with an additional environmental microphone on the receiver.

- Large area FM system for church members with hearing loss that attaches to the existing PA system

ON THE JOB WITH HEARING LOSS
Hearing Loss Issues and Retail Workers

The purpose of this report is to help you more fully identify potential communication barriers on the job. Each report focuses on a specific employment situation or topic and offers possible solutions to typical job functions. The combination of hearing instruments, assistive technology and communication strategies play a significant role in obtaining successful communication.

Retail Workers

People who work in retail store settings have several communication areas that are particularly difficult. These include knowing when a customer is asking for help and being able to respond to overhead pages. It is our experience that many store managers are willing to address the communication issues so that an employee can function as fully as possible.

Communication Demands of Typical Job Functions

- Hear and understand customers while out on the floor

- Hear customers at the cash register

- Respond to overhead pages

- Hear during staff meetings

- Understand clearly on the phone

Issues to Consider

Knowing when customers are asking for help is of primary importance. It's often difficult to hear a customer who is not facing the individual with hearing loss. Employees do not want to be perceived as rude or indifferent, yet they are unaware that someone is talking to them. This is a very difficult situation with no easy answers. Some employees have had buttons made that say "Please Face Me – I Read Lips" to instruct customers how to best communicate with them. Hearing instruments are the most important technology to help in this situation.

Hearing clearly at the checkout is also a difficult situation. The button mentioned before has also been helpful at the checkout (Please Face Me – I Read Lips). One communication strategy that is helpful for the individual with hearing loss is to repeat back to the customer what he or she thought they heard. Another strategy for the individual with hearing loss is to tell people how to talk to him or her.

An FM system can sometimes be used at the checkout. This is one of those creative solutions and usually involves the manager to help address how best to set-up the equipment. Basically, the transmitter with microphone is mounted on a pole or goose-neck stand so that the microphone is facing the customer. The cashier wears the receiver with appropriate listening option to better hear the customer.

Another option is a personal amplifier with a lapel microphone. The unit can stay in a pocket while the microphone is placed on the lapel to better pick up sound between the cashier and the customer. These have been used to supplement the hearing instrument to provide additional help when the environment is noisy.

Hearing overhead pages can be difficult. Many employees on the floor must be able to respond to overhead pages. Retail stores are notorious for incomprehensible announcements. Staff training on clear speech at a moderate pace can be helpful to employees and customers alike.

A push button paging system eliminates reliance on the audible signal by using a pager instead. The base transmitter sits at the customer service desk. The employee wears a pager-sized vibrating receiver. Codes are devised such as 1-to the front desk, 2-to receiving, etc. The person at the customer service desk simply enters the code and presses 'SEND'. The receiver will vibrate and display the code. This "Private Page" system requires no phone lines, no license and has a 1-2 mile radius. It costs less than $200.

Understanding when the page is for the employee can be difficult. Devising a name combined with numbers will alert the employee that the intercom is for him or her. James may miss the first word *"James* to the front" and not know it was for him. Adding the numbers '1' and '2' with a pause after the name may make it easier to identify. *"James 1 (short pause)*

2 *(pause), come to the front please"*. This change in the phrasing and timing may better help James know the page is for him.

Understanding clearly on the phone can be difficult. An inline telephone amplifier at the service desk or in the office is a quick, effective accommodation. In-line amplifiers work on most business telephones. If an employee must use different phones, then a portable strap-on amplifier may be more effective.

Staff meetings are required and can be difficult. Obvious strategies include arriving early and being positioned as close to the speaker as possible. If this isn't helpful, asking the speaker to follow-up on key points after the meeting can be arranged. If an FM system is used for other areas, then it can be used in this meeting as well.

Case Study

Jeff works at a retail store out on the floor, stocking shelves and helping customers. Jeff has a severe hearing loss and depends on speech-reading. On many occasions, Jeff has turned around to find a customer talking to him. He does not hear them come up or call out to him and he misses all that has been said. Oftentimes, the customer becomes frustrated with him.

Jeff feels that he appears rude and uncaring. He is very helpful once he is aware that someone is speaking to him. This scenario occurs every day and Jeff is becoming discouraged. He also misses overhead pages because he cannot tell that the page is for him.

The employer installed a private paging system with a vibrating receiver. Jeff wears the receiver and whenever someone needs to page him, they call the customer service desk. The paging transmitter sits at the customer service desk and a clerk will page Jeff using pre-determined codes to give instructions.

Jeff also uses a button on the back and front of his shirt that says, "Please face me, I read lips". He watches for visual cues that someone may be speaking to him. He is using a personal amplifier that he can face towards customers to help amplify their voice.

Jeff attends the daily meetings and stands near the front for the best visual cues possible.

Common Technical Accommodations

- Private Page paging system with vibrating receiver

- Personal amplifier (like PockeTalker)

- Name tag or button

- FM system with a transmitter/microphone and a receiver with a listening option that gets the sound to the hearing aid or to the ear

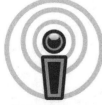

ON THE JOB WITH HEARING LOSS
Hearing Loss Issues and Teachers

The purpose of this report is to help you more fully identify potential communication barriers on the job. Each report focuses on a specific employment situation or topic and offers possible solutions to typical job functions. The combination of hearing instruments, assistive technology and communication strategies play a significant role in obtaining successful communication.

Teachers

Helping teachers hear more clearly in the classroom is one of the most challenging occupations to accommodate effectively. There is no one solution that will work for everyone.

Before offering a solution, it may be best to discuss many of the issues that face teachers and then take into consideration several important factors that will determine a workable solution.

Communication Demands of Typical Job Functions

- Hear students' questions
- Hear the aide or second teacher in the room
- Understand intercom messages
- Know when someone is at the door
- Hear the fire alarm
- Hear in staff meetings and parent meetings
- Hear on the telephone

Issues to Consider

Physical Classroom Environment – Can it be improved?

- Is the classroom self contained or is it an open shared area?
- Is there background noise that interferes in the classroom? Heating/air conditioning vents, fans, outside noise (traffic/construction)
- How is the classroom seating arranged? Are there individ-

ual desks in row seating, rectangular or circular tables? Can the room be rearranged?

- Is the classroom in a building or is it a mobile unit?
- Is there carpeting on the floor or rubber tips on the chairs?
- Is there an intercom system or telephone in the room?

Teacher's Hearing Aids or Cochlear Implants

- Telecoils on a hearing aid are helpful if the background noise is loud and an FM system is used. An M/T setting on the hearing aid may be most useful (microphone plus telecoil at the same time).
- Behind-the-Ear hearing aids with direct audio input will allow a wireless FM system to be used.
- Cochlear implant speech processors (both ear-level processors and body worn processors) have the capability to patch into an FM system. The options are based on the manufacturer and model.

Age of Students and Teaching Style

- There may be more movement and one-on-one discussions within the classroom in elementary school as well as more noise. Children's voices are higher pitched and/or softer in volume and thus more difficult to hear. Children may be more accepting of any technology the teacher uses (handheld may be preferred).
- Middle school and high school teachers sometimes have concerns about how the technology will be viewed by students. Some teachers do not want students to know what they are using and feel it could undermine their control.

Common Technical Accommodations

- Install an inline phone amplifier
- Mount a doorbell or door access monitor on the door to provide a signal to a wearable vibrating receiver. The receiver vibrates to alert the teacher that someone is at the door (like personal paging from Silent Call)
  - Deliver important intercom messages in writing to the teacher

or call them on the room phone.

- Add a visual smoke alarm in sight of the room. A phone call or another teacher can be assigned as backup for alarm notification.

- Place an FM remote microphone close to the students. The FM system can interface to the teacher's hearing aids allowing him or her to hear both the students and the room sounds.

FM Systems

An FM system will help provide a cleaner speech signal when there is distance from the speaker, reverberation in the room or background noise. Teachers can benefit the same way as students who use FM systems.

The <u>key</u> to an effective FM system <u>is the microphone placement</u>. Instead of one-to-one like a teacher to a student, the teacher needs a many-to-one configuration. FM systems operate on a radio frequency and only one transmitter can operate at a time on the same frequency so using several transmitters with microphones is not an option.

The <u>interface to the FM system</u> is limited to the teacher's hearing aid style. If the teacher has CIC or ITE hearing aids without telecoils, then the only options are an ear-hook or headphones. ITE or BTE hearing aids with telecoils can use a neckloop as a listening option. Only BTE hearing aids and cochlear implants can use direct audio input.

Using the telecoil may present a problem in that the hearing aid microphone is turned off and only sound coming through the FM system can be heard. This is a drawback when the teacher needs to monitor the classroom for other sounds as well. Some people will put one hearing aid on telecoil while keeping the hearing aid microphone turned on in the opposite ear.

The choice of the <u>appropriate FM system</u> should depend on the teacher's level of hearing loss and interface options to the FM system. A hearing professional should be able to recommend the most appropriate FM system for the individual's level of hearing loss.

FM System References

One of these types of FM systems may be recommended and the system configurations and benefits of each system follow this list:

- Wireless FM Systems (Microlink and Lexis are brand names)
- Traditional FM Systems (Comtek, Williams Sound, Phonic Ear)
- FM System with Microphone Mixer for up to 6 microphones

Wireless FM Systems (HandHeld Option 1)

Phonak Microlink

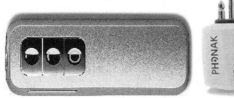

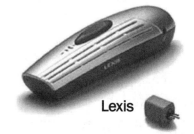

Lexis

Who Can Use the System

A wireless ear-level FM system like the Microlink or Lexis can be used if the hearing aids are BTE (behind-the-ear) style with the ability for direct audio input connection. Cochlear implant speech processors can also be interfaced to these systems.

The Microlink and Lexis systems operate on the 216 MHz frequencies and provide direct audio input into the hearing aid and will accommodate mild to profound hearing loss. The more severe the hearing loss and speech discrimination ability, the closer the transmitter (microphone) should be placed to the speakers mouth (handheld or lavaliere style).

System Components

The following items are needed to use this system: 1) a BTE hearing aid with direct audio input ability or appropriate interface to a cochlear implant speech processor 2) an audio shoe for the BTE aid (available from the audiologist to match the hearing aid) and 3) the transmitter with the ability for omni-directional, semi-directional or directional microphone settings.

How the System Works

The transmitter can be handheld, set on a table or worn around the neck. The receiver snaps onto an audio shoe of the hearing aid and permits three settings, hearing aid microphone only, FM system only or a combination of both.

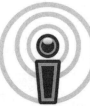

The ability to listen to both the FM system and the hearing aid microphone allows the listener to hear environmental sounds normally while also receiving sound from the transmitter.

The transmitter can be handheld as the teacher walks around the classroom. It can be passed around or mounted in one area. It can also be used in meetings. There are no specifications on the distance from the transmitter to the desired sound source because results can vary based on the individual's hearing loss and speech discrimination abilities.

Best Practical Use

This system is best used if students can pass around the microphone or if the teacher moves through the room while he or she teaches. If the teacher can hear the front of the room fairly well but not the back of the room, then the transmitter may be passed around by the students toward the back of the class.

For the Microlink and HandyMic (TX3) system: www.phonak.com/professional/productsp/fm/transmitters.htm

For the Lexis system: www.phonicear.com/PDFs/lxspec.pdf

Comtek FM System with Boom Microphone (HandHeld Option 2)

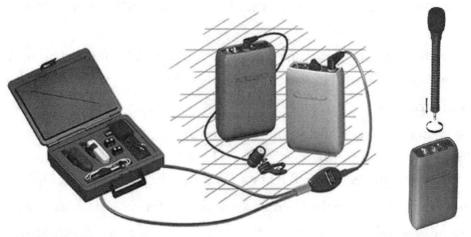

Comtek FM System with Boom Microphone on transmitter

Who Can Use the System

The Comtek AT216 FM system can be used by individuals with mild to profound hearing loss. Appropriate interfaces are available such as neckloop, DAI cables, cochlear implant cables, etc.

The Comtek systems operate on the 216 MHz frequencies. The more severe the hearing loss and speech discrimination ability, the closer the transmitter (microphone) should be placed to the speaker's mouth (handheld or lavaliere style).

System Components

The FM system consists of a transmitter with lapel microphone, conference microphone adapter, receiver with listening options, battery charger kit and case. The handheld boom microphone (COM-HH185) is also suggested for classroom use. The system can interface with hearing aids with telecoil option or cochlear implant speech processors.

How the System Works

The receiver directs sound to the hearing aid via a neckloop for aids with telecoils or with a cable for direct audio input. The receiver can also have an environmental microphone attached to be able to amplify sounds near the teacher (when speaking to an individual student).

The handheld boom microphone is suggested to use with the transmitter. The transmitter then can be used as a handheld microphone pointing towards a student (up to 8 feet away) or used as a pass around microphone. Results of the microphone pickup range can vary based on the individual's hearing loss and speech discrimination abilities.

The lapel microphone and conference microphone adapter can be used for small meetings when set in the center of the table.

Best Practical Use

This system is best used if students can pass around the microphone or if the teacher moves through the classroom. The teacher may be able to pick up sounds from students within 8 feet and can simply point the microphone.

For more information on the Comtek systems, see the manufacturer's website.

www.Comtek.com

Any FM System and Microphone Mixer (Remote Mic Option 1)

Who Can Use the System:

The Comtek AT216 FM system can be used by individuals with mild to profound hearing loss. Appropriate interfaces are available such as neckloop, DAI cables, cochlear implant cables, etc. The Phonic Ear and Williams Sound systems can be used for mild to moderate hearing loss.

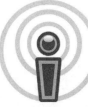

System Components

The FM system consists of a transmitter with lapel microphone, receiver with listening options, battery charger kit and case. The system can interface to hearing aids with telecoil option or cochlear implant speech processors.

The microphone mixer consists of a mixer and up to 6 omni-directional microphones with specific cable lengths of your choice.

How the System Works

The microphone mixer plugs into the microphone jack of the transmitter. It should be centrally located in the room. From that mixer, up to 6 cables with omni-directional microphones will branch out to different areas. The microphones can be worn or mounted, or conference microphones can be used in place of the lapel microphones.

The mixer enables the microphones to be placed strategically in the room. The conference microphones are designed to be placed on round or rectangular tables, not on individual desks.

Best Practical Use

This system will work best if the classroom does not change layouts. The cables will need to be secured so that students won't trip or arrange the desks/tables so that the cables won't run across the floor. This system gives the optimum in microphone placement.

This system can also be used for meetings by using the lapel or conference microphones.

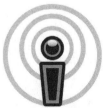

ON THE JOB WITH HEARING LOSS
Hearing Loss Issues and Truck Drivers

The purpose of this report is to help you more fully identify potential communication barriers on the job. Each report focuses on a specific employment situation or topic and offers possible solutions to typical job functions. The combination of hearing instruments, assistive technology and communication strategies play a significant role in obtaining successful communication.

Truck Drivers

Truck drivers with hearing loss have several unique communication obstacles to address. They must be able to hear their truck radio or cell phone in the presence of background noise. They must communicate with jobsite personnel and be able to hear abnormal truck operating sounds.

Communication Demands of Typical Job Functions

- Communicate with the dispatcher via radio or cellular phone
- Hear jobsite personnel when they pick up or deliver a load
- Monitor irregular truck operating sounds
- Attend company meetings
- Hear an alarm clock

Issues to Consider

Of all the technology available, hearing aids will offer the most significant improvement for this occupation.

The hearing aid will help the truck driver monitor irregular truck operating sounds. Additional technology might be needed to hear the radio clearly or to hear people at the jobsite because of background noise.

If the driver has severe hearing loss, then the hearing aid's options will become increasingly important so that the hearing aid will interface to other technology. The hearing aid telecoil with neckloop option provides an interface to work radios and cell phones.

Work radios and cell phones

It is critical to hear the work radio or the cell phone. There are cell phone accessories that will get the sound to the hearing aid's telecoil with an induction neckloop or directly to the hearing aid via direct audio input.

Noisy Communication Situations

An FM system is an assistive listening system. It can be used in the truck to monitor the radio, used at the jobsite if it is extremely noisy and used in all company meetings. The FM system is made up of two units. One is the FM transmitter/microphone that is placed next to the desired sound source (near the radio, on the presenter in a meeting). The second unit is the FM receiver that is worn by the truck driver. It has a listening option that gets the sound to the ear.

People with mild-to-moderate loss (and in-the-canal aids) may be able to use lightweight headphones or a single earphone to direct the sound to their ear. Depending on the level of hearing loss, these options may provide a good interface with the FM system without the hearing aids squealing.

If most communication is in very noisy situations, hearing aids may hinder instead of help understanding speech. The telecoil option on the hearing aids may overcome this challenge. The telecoil turns off the hearing aid's microphone so that only the sound through the FM system is picked up and amplified. The neckloop option on the FM receiver provides a clear signal to the hearing aid's telecoil.

Company meetings can be difficult, especially if the meetings are large. One option is to arrive early to find a seat in front or near the speaker. The use of an assistive listening system also provides a clear signal from the speaker to the person with hearing loss. If the individual is late deafened, then use CART reporting to provide real-time text. If the individual uses American Sign Language, use an interpreter.

Hearing an alarm clock

If the driver sleeps in the truck or in a hotel, they will need to hear the alarm clock. A loud alarm may not be much help if the truck engine is running. A vibrating alarm clock is useful for these situations. It should be battery powered and have means to secure it to the pillow or to a shirt pocket.

Case Study

John is an over-the-road truck driver. He has just found out he has a hearing loss and cannot maintain his CDL license unless he finds accommodations. In John's occupation, hearing aids are the primary technology that will help him in most all listening situations.

John sees an audiologist and describes his work situation, including how loud the truck engine is. Programmable hearing aids have been recommended and he may need to return to the hearing professional for fine-tuning adjustments so that he can hear best while in the truck.

John has trouble hearing the work radio/cell phone while driving. Hearing aids may help this situation but he may still have difficulty if the radio does not have a good speaker. He can use a special headset with the cell phone so that the sound goes directly to the hearing aid.

When John arrives on a jobsite, he must be able to hear the people there. There is a great deal of background noise at many of the locations and he has trouble hearing directions. If hearing aids do not provide enough benefit, he may find a personal amplifier helpful.

John sometimes naps in the truck if he arrives early to a jobsite. He needs to hear an alarm clock. To wake up, he clips a battery powered vibrating alarm clock to his shirt pocket.

Common Technical Accommodations

- A battery powered vibrating alarm clock (like the Shake Awake)
- Cell phone headset (like the T-Link silhouette) for hearing aids with telecoils
- FM System (like the Williams Sound Hearing Helper system)
- Text cell phones or text pager (like a Sidekick or Treo) if hearing on the phone is too difficult

Chapter 11 – Common Technical Accommodations

There are different types of products that can provide technical solutions. They are called assistive listening and alerting devices or hearing assistive technologies. Other services, including Remote Captioning or Interpreting services, use computer and telecommunication services and are also referenced here.

Technology changes and new products are introduced at a rapid pace. The products listed here should be used as reference. The products are representative of a wide array of manufacturers. **Inclusion of manufacturer products does not imply endorsement.**

The goal is to display technology that has been mentioned throughout the book and to offer direction and guidance for potential solutions.

- **Telephone Solutions**
- **Cell Phone Accessories**
- **Alerting Devices**
    - Telephones
    - Doorbells
    - Alarm Clocks
    - Emergency Alerting / Overhead Pages
- **Listening Situations**
    - Hearing at small meetings
    - Hearing at large meetings
    - Hearing from behind the counter
- **Specialized Equipment**
    - Stethoscopes
    - Dictation Equipment
    - Hearing Protection Headset
- **Specialized Technology**
    - Video Conferencing
    - VRI
    - CART

Telephone Solutions

It is best to use the existing work phone if possible to preserve all the features of the phone system.

Inline phone amplifier fits between the handset and base of the phone.

Headset amplifier fits between the handset and base of the phone. It accepts Plantronics headsets for CIC and ITE hearing aids.

The Hatis Headset can also work with the headset amplifier with a special adapter cord.

If it is not possible to hear on the phone clearly, use the Relay Service. Relay uses a special operator that provides text of the hearing caller 3 ways:

Voice Carry Over phone allows the hard of hearing person's voice to be heard by the other party.

TTY is a text telephone that provides text interface to Relay or to other TTY users.

Captel phone allows the hard of hearing person to read and listen to the caller.

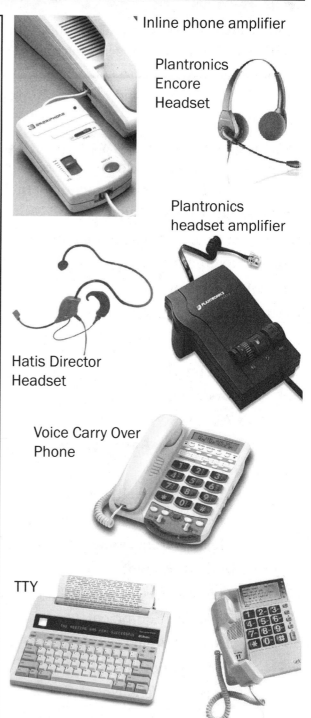

Inline phone amplifier

Plantronics Encore Headset

Plantronics headset amplifier

Hatis Director Headset

Voice Carry Over Phone

TTY

Captel Phone – Photo courtesy Ultratec

Cell Phone Accessories

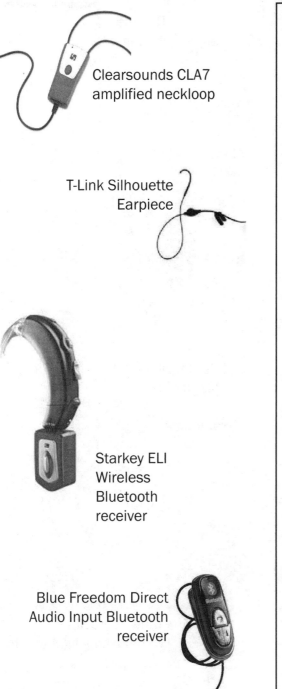

Clearsounds CLA7 amplified neckloop

T-Link Silhouette Earpiece

Starkey ELI Wireless Bluetooth receiver

Blue Freedom Direct Audio Input Bluetooth receiver

Plugs into DAI boot of BTE aid.

These accessories plug into the headset jack of the cell phone with 2.5mm round jack. Not all phones are compatible.

These three options use the tele-coil on any style hearing aid.

HATIS
T-LINK
Clearsounds Amplified
    Neckloop

These two options are Blue-tooth receivers for BTE hearing aids. They work with Bluetooth enabled cell phones and an audio boot for the hearing aid.

The ELI and the Blue Freedom plug into the audio boot of a BTE hearing aid to provide the connection.

(Watch for Bluetooth technology to explode with many more options)

Text Options
If unable to hear on the cell phone, use the cell phone speak-erphone as a last resort, or try a text device. The Blackberry and T-Mobile Sidekick are wireless text devices.

Many cell phones have text or email capability.

Alerting Devices

Telephones

Ringmax adjustable ringer changes the ring tones.

Alertmaster AM100 phone/door signaler uses a lamp that you plug into it for alerting.

Telestrobe industrial phone signaler (not pictured).

Ringmax
adjustable ringer

Alertmaster
AM100

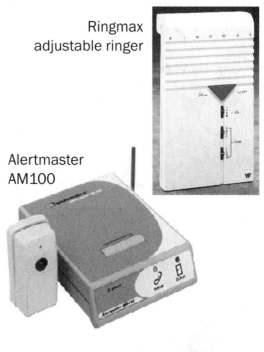

Doorbells

Alertmaster signaler causes lamp to flash for phone or doorbell ring.

Magnetic access transmitter and vibrating receiver can alert you to a door opening.

Doorbell with flashing strobe light. Plug the chime/strobe receiver where you can see it.

Silent Call
Magnetic
Access
Transmitter

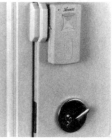

Trine doorbell
with flashing light and tone

Photo courtesy Harris Communications

Alerting Devices – Continued

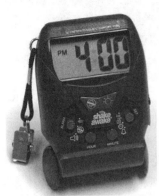

Shake-Awake

Vibrating Alarm Clocks

Shake Awake portable clock

Sonic Boom alarm clock

AM6000 for travel use (not shown)

Sonic Boom Vibrating Alarm Clock

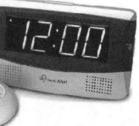

Emergency Signaling System

Private Page System (see below)

Fire alarm transmitter and Omni Page receiver or strobe light

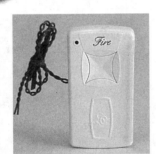

Silent Call Omni Page receiver and fire alarm transmitter

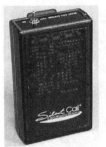

Private Page Base Transmitter

Overhead Pages

Private Page System

Email to text pager or cell phone (not shown)

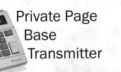

Private Page Vibrating Receiver

Photos courtesy Harris Communications

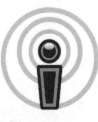

Listening Situations

Hearing at small meetings

An FM system like the one pictured will allow an individual to hear around the table with the use of conference microphones.

Phonak offers a miniaturized receiver that can plug into BTE hearing aids. These offer true wireless capability. They have several transmitters with directional microphones that will work in small and medium group settings.

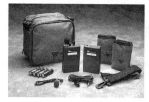

Williams Sound FM System with environmental microphone.

Centrum Sound conference microphone

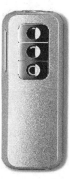

Phonak Microlink receiver and Smartlink transmitter

The Companion Mic System from Etymotic Research is a promising system for anyone who regularly attends small group meetings with 3-4 people.

It allows each 'talker' to wear their own microphone transmitter and the 'listener' to wear a receiver that can pick up all 4 transmitters simultaneously.

The benefit is the ability to place a microphone on each speaker to get the best signal to noise ratio possible.

Coypright: Etymotic Research, Inc.

Used with permission

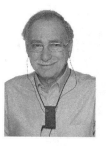

Companion Mic System

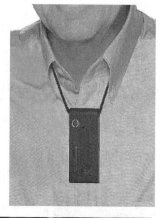

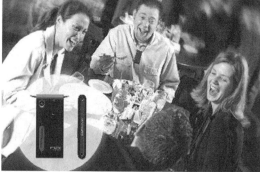

Listening Situations - Continued

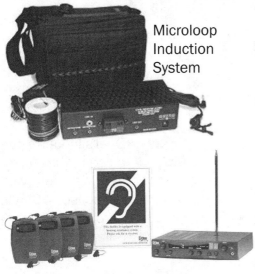

Microloop Induction System

Listen Large Area FM System

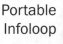

Portable Infoloop

PockeTalker Ultra Personal amplifier with earhook

Hearing at medium and large meetings

To make a large area accessible, using an FM system connected to an existing PA system will provide clear sound.

An induction loop system is another way to make meeting rooms accessible to people who wear hearing aids with telecoils. The benefit is receivers are only needed for those without hearing aids with telecoils.

Hearing From Behind a Counter or Desk

The Portable InfoLoop is placed on the counter with a forward facing microphone and creates a signal for the hearing aid telecoils of the person with hearing loss.

Use an FM system with microphone facing out.

A personal amplifier like the PockeTalker Ultra amplifier designed for one-on-one and small group listening situations. The amplifier has an external microphone to pick up sounds that are close. The listening option is chosen based on the hearing aids.

Specialized Equipment

Amplified Stethoscope Solutions

Cardionics manufactures amplified stethoscopes designed for hearing aid users.

There are several listening options available depending on hearing aid options.

CIC and ITE hearing aids can use the headphones.

ITE or BTE hearing aids with tele-coils can use the silhouette earpieces.

BTE hearing aids and **Cochlear Implant processors** with direct audio input can use special cables.

Aviation style headphones provide hearing protection and interface to an amplified stethoscope for EMS pesronnel.

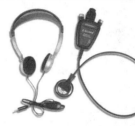

Cardionics Belt Clip amplified stethoscope. Shown with headphones.

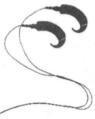

Dual silhouette ear-pieces shown for hearing aids with telecoils. Single earpiece also available.

Hearing Aid Audio Boot

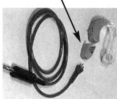

This is a direct audio input cable that will plug into the audio boot of the hearing aid. It snaps onto the hearing aid.

Cardionics amplified stethoscope with personal digital assistant (PDA) for visual representation.

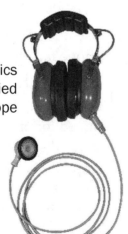

Cardionics EMS amplified stethoscope

Learning software available.

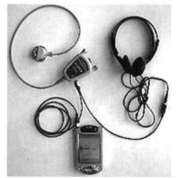

Specialized Equipment – Continued

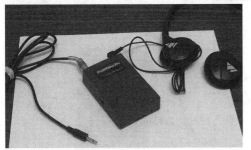

Products shown are Williams Sound auxiliary cable WCA040, Pocketalker Pro amplifier and headphones.

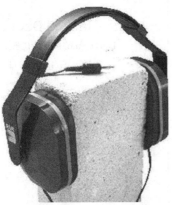

Williams Sound hearing protection headset HED008.

Williams Sound PockeTalker Ultra personal amplifier.

Dictation/Transcription Equipment

A dictation/transcription device must have a 3.5mm headset jack (or adapters are needed). Many of the systems are using pin connections and no adapters are available.

For amplification, a personal amplifier can be connected to the dictation equipment with an auxiliary cable. The preferred listening option can then be used (headphones, neckloop, direct audio input).

Hearing Protection Headset

If communication is necessary, this headset uses a cable to connect to a personal amplifier for one-on-one communication. When you turn off the amplifier, full hearing protection returns.

Another style electronic hearing protection headset uses forward facing microphones on the earcups.

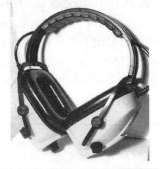

Specialized Equipment – Continued

Tactaid – Little Tactaid Device

This unit was primarily developed for speech training for individuals who are deaf. The microphones have a sensitivity switch that can be adjusted to pick up sounds around an individual.

Training is critical to the success of this unit. A hearing person should work with the deaf individual to identify sounds in the background. The deaf individual can then learn which vibrations indicate a specific sound.

This unit may be helpful in a warehouse setting, depending on the background noises. Please note that training is essential to understand the correlation of the vibration to the background sounds.

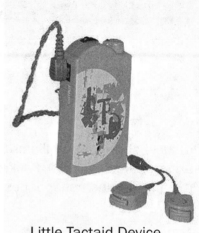

Little Tactaid Device from Audiological Engineering Corp

Specialized Technology

Audio Conference Telephones

Several high performance conference telephones are helpful to people with hearing loss. While the output from the conference speakers can be loud, it is important that other callers speak clearly into a microphone for best sound pick-up.

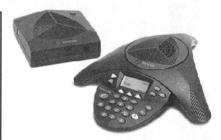

Polycom SoundStation2W Conference Telephone

photo courtesy Harris Communications

Specialized Technology - Continued

Video relay service (VRS)

VRS is important to people who prefer to use American Sign Language (ASL) to communicate. Video relay services can be accessed by using a high-speed or broadband internet connection (DSL or T1 line) and a video-phone connected to a TV, or by using video conferencing software like Microsoft NetMeeting, a computer monitor, web camera and special software.

The deaf or hard of hearing individual communicates with the relay operator who is a sign language interpreter by using the TV or monitor. The ASL user will communicate directly with the interpreter for a more natural and free flowing conversation while the interpreter speaks to the hearing caller. This service provides visual communication instead of text communication.

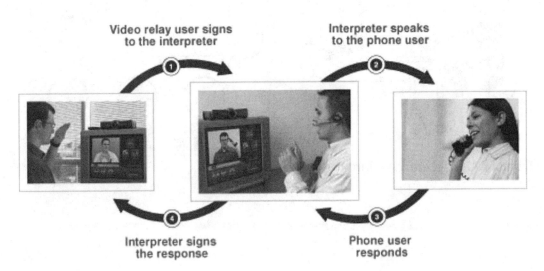

Video relay user signs to the interpreter

Interpreter speaks to the phone user

Interpreter signs the response

Phone user responds

Sorenson VRS - Used with permission

Specialized Technology - Continued

Computer Access Real-time Translation (CART)

The National Court Reporters Association (NCRA) definition of CART:

Communication Access Real-time Translation (CART) is the instant translation of the spoken word into English text using a stenotype machine, notebook computer and real-time software. The text appears on a computer monitor or other display. People who are late deafened, oral deaf, hard-of-hearing, or who have cochlear implants primarily use CART. Culturally deaf individuals also make use of CART in certain situations. Please keep in mind that CART is often referred to as real-time captioning.

Companies have evolved who offer remote CART when a CART reporter is not available locally.

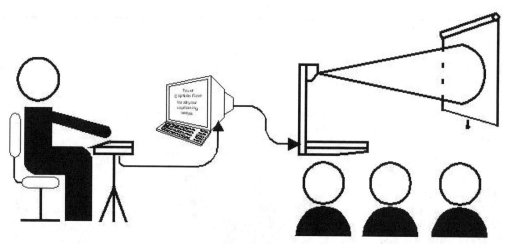

Typical CART set-up for a larger group meeting.
Used with permission: Caption First   www.captionfirst.com

Chapter 12 – Where to Get Help Resources

After reading this book, you may have even more questions or are interested in more information on topics not covered in-depth. This list will be maintained online at the author's website at www.beyondhearingaids.com.

- Employment Services and Higher Education Resources
- Individual and Family Training Programs
- National Hearing Healthcare Organizations
- Non-Profit Organizations
- Consumer Organizations and Personal Informational Websites
- Cochlear Implant Websites
- Telecommunications, Captioning and Video Relay Services
- Recommended Reading

Employment Services and Higher Education Resources

American with Disabilities (ADA) Homepage
Website:www.usdoj.gov/crt/ada/adahom1.htm
Information and technical assistance on the ADA

Website: www.usdoj.gov/crft/ada/taxpack.htm
A packet of information is available to help businesses understand and take advantage of the tax credits and deductions available for complying with the ADA.

Business Leadership Network
Website: www.usbln.com

The US Business Leadership Network (USBLN) is the national organization that supports development and expansion of BLNs across the country, serving as their collective voice. The USBLN recognizes and promotes best practices in hiring, retaining, and marketing to people with disabilities.

State chapters exist and contact information about local chapters can be found through the website.

Council of State Administrators of Vocational Rehabilitation

CSAVR is a membership organization of the Directors of the 80 vocational rehabilitation programs across the country, in the territories (such as Guam and Puerto Rico) and in the District of Columbia.

Website: www.rehabnetwork.org

EARN

Website: www.earnworks.com

Today's employers are competing for job applicants in many fields. As a result, employers are searching for qualified workers and have begun to explore "non-traditional" labor pools such as people with disabilities. EARN helps you tap into this labor pool.

EARN is a free service expanding the creative ways that employers meet the growing challenge of finding talented, motivated, and dedicated workers for a full range of jobs.

EARN reaches out to an expansive network of recruiting sources, including Social Security beneficiaries ready to return to work through the Ticket to Hire program, advocacy groups, vocational rehabilitation agencies, and colleges and universities.

An EARN employment specialist will also answer questions about disability employment, including legal issues, accommodations, disability etiquette and more.

Job Accommodation Network

The Job Accommodation Network is a service of the Office of Disability Employment Policy (ODEP) of the U.S. Department of Labor. JAN is one of several ODEP projects. JAN's mission is to provide a free consulting service designed to increase the employability of people with disabilities by 1) providing individualized worksite accommodations solutions, 2) providing technical assistance regarding the ADA and other disability related legislation, and 3) educating callers about self employment options.

PO Box 608, Morgantown, WV 26506-6080

Telephone: 800-526-7234 (V/TTY) in the United States
Website: www.jan.wvu.edu

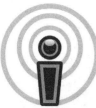

Vocational Rehabilitation Services

Each state has an agency or department with vocational rehabilitation counselors who provide assistance to eligible individuals with hearing loss to help them obtain, retain and maintain employment. You should be able to find local information by looking in the phone book under the government/state section for Vocational Rehabilitation or Rehabilitation Services. The link below of state agencies contact information is maintained by JAN, the Job Accommodation Network:

Website: www.jan.wvu.edu/SBSES/VOCREHAB.HTM

PEPNet, the Postsecondary Education Programs Network

A national collaboration of the four Regional Postsecondary Education Centers for Individuals who are Deaf and Hard of Hearing. The Centers are supported by contracts with the U.S. Department of Education, Office of Special Education and Rehabilitative Services. The goal of PEPNet is to assist postsecondary institutions across the nation to attract and effectively serve individuals who are Deaf and Hard of Hearing.

Website: www.pepnet.org

Workforce Recruitment Program

The 2006 Workforce Recruitment Program database containing profiles of student job candidates is now available. Fill your summer or permanent hiring needs with talented college students with disabilities. These candidates, from more than 200 colleges and universities, represent all majors, and range from college freshmen to graduate students and law students. To request a free copy of the entire WRP database on CD-ROM, send your name, company name and mailing address to wrp@dol.gov. Please note: if you represent a federal agency, contact wrp@dol.gov for information on access to the WRP.

Program Description: Coordinated by the Office of Disability Employment Policy and the U.S. Department of Defense, the Workforce Recruitment Program aims to provide summer work experience, and in some cases full-time employment, for college students with disabilities. The program develops partnerships with other federal agencies, each of whom makes a commitment to provide summer jobs and a staff recruiter.

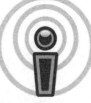

U.S. Department of Labor
Frances Perkins Building
200 Constitution Avenue, NW
Washington, DC 20210
Telephone: 866-633-7365
Website: www.dol.gov/odep/programs/workforc.htm

Individual and Family Training Programs

The Living with Hearing Loss Program

Dr. Trychin's **Living With Hearing Loss Program** is a product of twenty-two years of experience working directly with hundreds of people who are hard of hearing and their family members. Additionally, many more people who are hard of hearing, their family members, and professionals who serve them have benefited from his training programs, presentations, and workshops.

Hearing loss is a communication disorder affecting everyone in the communication situation-- the person speaking as well as the person with hearing loss who is trying to listen. For that reason, the **Living With Hearing Loss Program** is designed to meet the needs of family members, friends, coworkers, and service providers as well as the person who is hard of hearing.

Website: www.trychin.com

The Kooser Program

Cathy Kooser-Fathergill, MSW

The Kooser Program is an aural rehabilitation program available nationwide to hearing healthcare professionals. These professionals may work in conjunction with their vocational rehabilitation agencies to provide the program to their consumers with hearing loss. The goal of the program is to improve the quality of life of persons with hearing loss by empowerment through education and support services. The program is 12 hours and seeks to educate the person with hearing loss as well as their loved ones regarding the psychosocial impact of this disability. They teach positive coping skills and communication strategies and discuss many pertinent issues including hearing loss in the workplace.

Website: www.thekooserprogram.com

Cochlear Implant Websites

Advanced Bionics Corporation
12740 San Fernando Rd.
Smylar, CA 91342
Telephone: 800-678-2575
Email: info@advancedbionics.com
Website: www.bionicear.com

Cochlear Corporation
400 Inverness Parkway, Suite 400
Englewood, CO 80112
Telephone: 800-523-5798
Email: info@cochlear.com
Website: www.cochlear.com

MED-EL Corporation (North America)
2222 East Highway 54
Beta Building, Suite 180
Durham, NC 27713
Telephone: 888-633-3524
Email: implants@medelus.com
Website: www.medel.com

National Hearing Healthcare Organizations

Academy of Dispensing Audiologists
The ADA is dedicated to leadership in advancing practitioner excellence, high ethical standards, professional autonomy, hearing technology, and sound business practices in the provision of quality audiological care. Provides a useful consumer information section.

PO Box 15056
Asheville, NC 28813
Telephone: 866-493-5544
Website: www.audiologist.org

Audiologist Awareness Campaign

Information is provided from five professional organizations to consumers. Questionnaires to help measure the amount of problems a person might be having in daily situations that may be caused by hearing loss. The Hearing Help Library stores current consumer information about hearing, hearing loss, hearing aids, and other audiology related areas.

Website: www.audiologyawareness.com

American Academy of Audiology

The American Academy of Audiology (AAA) is a professional organization for Audiologists. Provides a useful consumer information section.

11730 Plaza America Dr., Suite 300
Reston, VA 20190
Telephone: 800.AAA.2336
Website:_   www.audiology.org

American Speech-Language-Hearing Association

The American Speech-Language-Hearing Association (ASHA) is the professional, scientific and credentialing association for audiologists, speech-language pathologists, and speech, language and hearing scientists. Provides good public consumer information.

10801 Rockville Pike
Rockville, MD 20852
Telephone: 800-638-8255
Website: www.asha.org

International Hearing Society

The non-profit professional association that represents Hearing Instrument Specialists worldwide. As the membership organization for thousands of independent specialists, IHS conducts programs in competency accreditation, education and training and promotes specialty-level certification for its members.

Website: www.ihsinfo.org

Non-Profit Organizations

American Tinnitus Association

We help people with ringing in the ears. We also help people who hear whooshing or buzzing or chirping or pulsing. We help people who have tinnitus, the perception of noise in the ears or head when no external sound is present.

PO Box 5
Portland, OR 97207
Telephone: 800-634-8978
Website: www.ata.org

Association of Medical Professionals With Hearing Losses (AMPHL)

A non-profit online organization that provides information, promotes advocacy and mentorship, and creates a network for individuals with hearing loss interested in or working in health care fields.

Website: www.amphl.org

Audient Program

Nationwide program providing assistance to low income hearing impaired seniors, children and families. Helping them access quality hearing aids and related hearing care at a significantly lower cost.

901 Boren Ave., Ste 810
Seattle, WA 98104-3534
Telephone: 877-283-4368
Website: www.audientalliance.org

Better Hearing Institute

BHI's goal is to educate the public about the neglected problem of hearing loss and what can be done about it. For example, thanks to BHI, nearly 60 Hollywood celebrities, sports personalities, business leaders and other noteworthy Americans have come forward to share their stories about hearing loss and how they have addressed it.

515 King Street, Suite 420
Alexandria, VA 22314
Telephone: 703-684-3391
Website: www.betterhearing.org

The EAR Foundation

The EAR Foundation's mission is to enrich the lives of the hearing and balance impaired through public awareness and continuing medical education.

PO Box 330867
Nashville, TN 37203
Telephone: 1-800-545-HEAR
Website: www.earfoundation.org

Hearing Education and Awareness for Rockers

H.E.A.R. is a non-profit organization dedicated to educating the public on the dangers of excessive noise from music and promoting awareness of hearing damage.

H.E.A.R. Office (direct inquiries via phone or through website)
San Francisco, CA 94115
Telephone: 415-409-3277 10am-7pm PST
Website: www.hearnet.com

House Ear Institute

Non-profit organization with a comprehensive online library devoted to issues of the human auditory and related systems for use by both the general public and scientists and physicians. It has excellent graphics on "HOW WE HEAR".

2100 W. 3rd Street
Los Angeles, CA 90057
Telephone: (800) 388-8612
Website:_   www.hei.org

Hyperacusis Network

The Hyperacusis Network consists of individuals who have a collapsed tolerance to sound. Rich resources for people with hyperacusis.

PO Box 8007
Green Bay, WI 54308
Website: www.hyperacusisnetwork.net

National Acoustic Neuroma Association

We are a patient member organization, providing information and support to persons diagnosed with or treated for acoustic neuroma and other benign tumors of the cranial nerves.

600 Peachtree Pkwy. Suite 108
Cumming, GA 30041
Telephone: 877-200-8211
Website: www.anausa.org

National Association of the Deaf

The mission of NAD is to promote, protect and preserve the rights and quality of life of deaf and hard of hearing individuals in the U.S.

Website: www.nad.org

National Center for Hearing Assessment and Management

The goal of the National Center for Hearing Assessment and Management (NCHAM - pronounced "en-cham") at Utah State University is to ensure that all infants and toddlers with hearing loss are identified as early as possible and provided with timely and appropriate audiological, educational, and medical intervention.

2880 Old Main Hill
Logan, UT 84322
Telephone: 435-797-3584
Website: www.infanthearing.org

National Hearing Conservation Association

The mission of the NHCA is to prevent hearing loss due to noise and other environmental factors in all sectors of society. Our newly enhanced website is intended to provide information to anyone interested in learning more about hearing loss prevention.

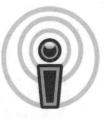

7995 E. Prentice Ave., Suite 100
Greenwood Village, CO 80111-2710
Telephone: 303-224-9022
Website: www.hearingconservation.org

National Institute on Deafness and other Communication Disorders

The National Institute on Deafness and Other Communication Disorders (NIDCD) is one of the Institutes that comprise the National Institutes of Health (NIH). NIH is the Federal government's focal point for the support of biomedical research. NIH's mission is to uncover new knowledge that will lead to better health for everyone. Simply described, the goal of NIH research is to acquire new knowledge to help prevent, detect, diagnose, and treat disease and disability. NIH is part of the U.S. Department of Health and Human Services.

National Institute on Deafness and Other Communication Disorders
National Institutes of Health
31 Center Drive, MSC 2320
Bethesda, MD 20892-2320
Telephone: 301-496-7243 (voice) 301-402-0252 (tty)
Website: www.nidcd.nih.gov

Telecommunications Equipment Distribution Program

TEDPA is a national membership organization formed to support programs involved in Statewide, or jurisdiction-wide, distribution of specialized telecommunications equipment for persons who have disabilities. It provides an online link for consumers to available programs in each state. Internet based for consumers.

Website: www.tedpa.org

Transportation Security Administration

For specific information and tips from the TSA for travelers, go to the public page and click on Travelers & Consumers. Then Choose: Persons with Disabilities and Medical Conditions and then Hearing Disabilities. Online resource.

Website: www.tsa.gov/public

Consumer Organizations and Other Informational Websites

Alexander Graham Bell Association

International membership organization and resource center on hearing loss and spoken language approaches and related issues. Publishes and distributes books, brochures and other materials related to hearing loss.

Website: www.agbell.org

Association of Late Deafened Adults

ALDA provides a support network and a sense of belonging for late deafened people and members help one another find practical solutions and psychological relief. ALDA publishes a newsletter, supports local and regional chapters and organizes an annual educational and networking conference.

Website: www.alda.org

Captioned Media Program

The Captioned Media Program is administered by The National Association of the Deaf (NAD) whose mission is to provide all persons who are deaf or hard of hearing awareness of and equal access to communication and learning through the use of captioned educational media and supportive collateral materials. The ultimate goal of the CMP is to permit media to be an integral part in the lifelong learning process for all stakeholders in the deaf and hard of hearing community: adults, students, parents, and educators.

National Association of the Deaf, CMP
1447 E. Main Street
Spartanburg, SC 29307
Telephone: 800-237-6213 (VOICE); 800-237-6819 (TTY)
Website: www.cfv.org

Digicare Research and Rehabilitation

The Digicare Hearing Health Network is a worldwide network of hearing health professionals dedicated to auditory research and rehabilitation. They develop practice models of patient care for the industry on various hearing health issues, such as hearing loss, tinnitus, cognitive dis-

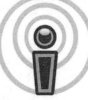

orders, and multidisciplinary approaches to healthcare. The exhaustive library of articles for consumers and professionals by Max Stanley Chartrand is the highlight of this website.

Website: www.digicare.org

Hearing Exchange

A supportive online community for people with hearing loss, parents of deaf and hard of hearing children and professionals who work with them. It provides an open forum for the discussion of ideas and information on hearing loss and features forums and chats.

HearingExchange.com
div. of Taylor Rose, Inc.
PO Box 689
Jericho, NY 11753
Website: www.hearingexchange.com

Hearing Loss Association of America

HLAA (formerly Self Help for Hard of Hearing People) is a national organization for people with hearing loss. HLAA exists to open the world of communication for people with hearing loss through information, education, advocacy and support.

7910 Woodmont Ave., Suite 1200
Bethesda, MD 20814
Telephone: 301-657-2248
Website: www.hlaa.org

HearingLossHelp.com

A website with very easy to read and understand information. Articles and materials are written by Neil Bauman, Ph.D. a hearing loss coping skills specialist, researcher, author and speaker on issues pertaining to hearing loss.

49 Piston Court
Stewartstown, PA 17363-8322
Telephone: 717-993-8555
      Website: www.hearinglosshelp.com

Recommended Reading

Baby Boomers and Hearing Loss – A Guide to Prevention and Care
By John M. Burkey

This book explains why baby boomers should be concerned about hearing loss and how to preserve their hearing. It presents techniques, equipment and medical procedures that can benefit a person with hearing loss. It also discusses unresolved hearing care issues that are a concern to baby boomers.

The Consumer Handbook on Hearing Loss and Hearing Aids
Edited by Clinical Audiologist Richard Carmen, Au.D. Doctor of Audiology

Topics include exploring volatile emotions and issues of hearing loss, how to map your own audiogram, ways to improve your quality of life, questions and answers posed to 10 top experts, master incredibly easy techniques to improve your listening and hearing ability.

Hearing Instrument Counseling: Practical Applications for Counseling the Hearing Impaired
By Max S. Chartrand

Text book for the International Institute for Hearing Instrument Studies, 1999 edition.

How Hearing Loss Impacts Relationships—Motivating Your Loved One
By Richard Carmen, Au.D, Doctor of Audiology

Topics include understanding feelings, establishing a framework for help, discussing whose problem it is, consequences of untreated hearing loss and solutions. This book is filled with helpful tips for families living with a loved one resistant to help.

Website: www.hearingproblems.com

Legal Rights: The Guide for Deaf and Hard of Hearing People
By DuBow, S., Geer, S., Peltz Strauss, K. Washington, DC: Gallaudet Press

A comprehensive analysis of recent laws passed to protect the rights of and guarantee equal access for people with hearing loss. In this revised, fifth edition, the book explains in layman's terminology how legislation affects individuals with disabilities in everyday life.

Living with Hearing Loss

By Marcia Dugan

Written in collaboration with SHHH. Foreword by Rocky Stone, founder of SHHH. People who are hard of hearing and their friends and family can learn all they need to know about hearing loss in this easy-to-read guide. Newly updated and revised, Living with Hearing Loss takes the reader from A to Z on the kinds and causes of hearing loss and its common early signs. Topics Include: Seeking Professional Evaluations, Hearing Aids, Assistive Technology, Speechreading, Communication Tips, Cochlear Implants, Dealing with Tinnitus, and Resources.

Telecommunications, Captioning and Video Relay Services

AT & T Video Relay Service
Website: www.consumer.att.com/relay/video/

Caption First
The primary goal of Caption First is to provide real-time captioning (CART) services at many different events including counseling sessions, meetings, teleconferences, seminars, classrooms and conventions.

Phone: (800) 825-5234

Website: www.captionfirst.com

Computer Access Real-time Translation (CART)
The primary purpose of the Communication Access Information Center is to provide information of use to people employing or in need of Communication Access Real-time Translation (CART), also known as real-time captioning. The site is sponsored by the National Court Reporters Foundation and supported by the National Court Reporters Association's CART Task Force.

Website: www.cartinfo.org

Federal Video Relay Service
Toll Free: (866)377-8642
TTY: (800)877-8339
Website: www.fedvrs.us/

Hands On Video Relay Service, Inc. (HOVRS)
Toll Free: (877)467-4877

Website: http://secure.hovrs.com/vrs_ssl/hovrs.aspx

Sorenson VRS
Sorenson Video Relay Service (VRS) is a free service for the deaf and hard-of-hearing community that enables anyone to conduct video relay calls with family, friends, or business associates through a certified ASL interpreter via a high-speed Internet connection and a video relay solution (or VRS call option).

4393 South Riverboat Road, Suite 300
Salt Lake City, UT 84123
Toll Free: (801)287-9400
Website: www.sorensonvrs.com

Sprint Video Relay Service
Website: www.sprintvrs.com

Index

About the Author

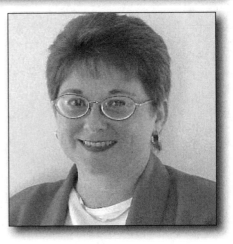

Becky Morris is the president of Beyond Hearing Aids, Inc., a company offering sales and services to professionals who recommend or purchase assistive listening and alerting devices. Her company serves vocational rehabilitation counselors, hearing health care professionals, disability services providers in post-secondary education and human resource managers in small and large companies.

The company website, www.beyondhearingaids.com, also offers products to consumers from their online store.

Becky has toured medium and maximum security facilities to understand the environment for corrections officers, climbed into heavy equipment, farm tractors and semi trucks, donned sterile gowns to observe inside hospital operating rooms and has toured factories, warehouses, call centers and innumerable office settings. Her unique perspective and 14+ years experience will help anyone trying to accommodate an employee with hearing loss.

She is a published author, a national and international presenter at professional conferences and recognized leader in ALDs in both hearing healthcare industry as well as the Vocational Rehabilitation arena. The company provides communication assessment services and training to professionals who work with people who have hearing loss.

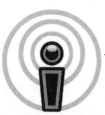

Communication Worksheet and Assessment Service

Who Uses the Communication Assessment Service?

Vocational rehabilitation counselors and employers find a Communication Assessment service valuable for case documentation. Counselors unfamiliar with all the issues surrounding someone who is hard of hearing find the service invaluable in helping them choose the most appropriate accommodations to meet their client's needs.

Even seasoned counselors find the information in the assessment helpful when dealing with complicated communication issues. It has been useful in providing third party recommendations to employers or documentation in a case.

Counselors who must choose clients based on order of selection find the assessment process helpful in the identification and documentation of the level of disability and impact the hearing loss has on successful employment outcomes, maintaining current employment and independent living.

Benefits of the Assessment Process:

- Gathering information in a systematic way ensures you obtain all the information in the same manner each time.
- Saves time by getting all the information the first time.
- Provides case documentation to help counselors save time.
- Functional and technical needs can be identified thoroughly and comprehensively.

How to Request the Communication Assessment Service

The process is simple. Use our Assessment Form for your employee to fill in and fax it to us with their audiological report, type of hearing aids and your case notes. We will prepare a comprehensive 5-page report for case management and documentation.

The tool itself, The Communication Questionnaire, is available free for your use, whether or not you need the assessment reporting service.

Communication Questionnaire

Instructions for the Client

- Please write or print clearly with a pen.
- Take your time answering these questions with as much detail as possible.
- Add comments, especially if you are having extra trouble in any area.
- Try to answer all of the questions that you can, don't skip any.
- *Return this questionnaire to your counselor.*

Instructions for the Counselor (if you want a formal evaluation and report)

- **IMPORTANT** --- review this questionnaire before sending it to make sure it is complete.
- Add any comments or insights that you may have.
- Include a recent audiogram and hearing aid evaluation report.

Mail to:	**Fax to:**
Beyond Hearing Aids, Inc.	859-371-1363
P. O. Box 353	
Florence, KY 41022-0353	

Purpose for this questionnaire

Hearing aids offer a tremendous improvement to hearing in everyday situations. However, hearing aids alone are not always enough when you face a difficult listening situation. There are products called assistive devices that can enhance the benefits of your hearing aids and improve the areas that you find difficult.

All the information you provide is used to help evaluate which technology will work most effectively for you. *That is why it is critical that both you and your counselor provide as much information as possible.*

All information contained herein is strictly confidential.

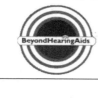

Beyond Hearing Aids, Inc.
P.O. Box 353, Florence, KY 41022-0353
1-800-838-1649 v/tty 859-371-1363 Fax
www.BeyondHearingAids.com

7/25/06

Communication Questionnaire

Today's Date_____ Audiogram Attached ☐

Client Information:

Name _____ Date of Birth _____

Address _____

City _____ State _____ Zip _____

Daytime Phone No. _____ Evening Phone No. _____

Email Address _____

If we have questions, may we contact you directly? _____

Referred by _____ Counselor _____

How do you most often communicate?	How would you describe your overall hearing loss without hearing aids?
___ Sign language	___ Mild ___ Severe
___ Fingerspelling	___ Mild to moderate ___ Severe to profound
___ Speaking and listening	___ Moderate ___ Profound
___ Speechreading & lip reading	___ Moderate to severe ___ Don't know
___ Tell people how to talk to me	

Please answer the following miscellaneous questions

When was your last audiogram?_____

Age you began noticing your hearing loss? _____

Do you have vision problems?_____

Do you live alone or with others? (please list)_____

Do you live in a: ☐House ☐Condo ☐Apartment ☐Mobile Home ☐Dorm

How many floors are in the house or condo?_____

Do you have a working doorbell? ☐Yes ☐No

Have you used any products that have been helpful to you?_____

Beyond Hearing Aids, Inc.
P.O. Box 353, Florence, KY 41022-0353
1-800-838-1649 v/tty 859-371-1363 Fax
www.BeyondHearingAids.com

On The Job With Hearing Loss

Please describe your experiences with hearing aids

Please check the statement that best describes your situation:

☐ I do not own a hearing aid and I am interested in finding out if one can help me.

☐ I owned a hearing aid at one time but don't use it now because:

    ☐ I felt the aid was physically uncomfortable

    ☐ I did not know how to operate or maintain the aid

    ☐ I did not find the aid very helpful

☐ I own a hearing aid and use it: (mark how often you use the hearing aid)
    ☐ All day, every day   ☐ Off and on during the day   ☐ Only on special occasions

☐ I would use my hearing aid more often if... (write in ways you think the aid could work better for you): _____

_____

Check the type of hearing aids or cochlear implant you use: ☐ Programmable   ☐ Digital

    ☐ Behind-the-ear (BTE)   ☐ In-the-ear (ITE)
    ☐ Completely-in-the-Canal (CIC)   ☐ Eyeglass or body aid
    ☐ Body worn speech processor   ☐ Ear level speech processor

---

Left Ear	**Right Ear**
Make and model: _____	Make and model: _____
Age of aid: _____	Age of aid: _____
☐ Telecoil ☐ Direct audio input	☐ Telecoil ☐ Direct audio input

Please tell us how you use the phone with your hearing aid or cochlear implant

Do you use your hearing aids with: *the telephone?* ☐ Yes ☐ No *the cell phone?* ☐ Yes ☐ No

If No, Explain why not _____

If Yes, Do you:

        ☐ Use the "T" switch (telecoil or telephone switch)?

        ☐ Hold the phone receiver next to the hearing aid microphone?

        ☐ Does the phone squeal when you use it this way?   ☐ Yes   ☐ No

Communication Questionnaire

Please tell us about work   I work   ☐Full time   ☐Part time

Occupation and Employer _____

I travel overnight for my job _____ nights a month

List your major job duties and describe any problems you have:

_____

_____

_____

_____

_____

Describe in detail how hard it is to communicate with the following people and include notes if background noise is a problem

Supervisor: _____

_____

_____

Co-workers: _____

_____

_____

Customers: _____

_____

_____

List any other areas that are difficult for you (including fire alarms, 2-way radios or other specialized equipment – you must include brand name of equipment)

_____

_____

_____

Is hearing protection required on the job? _____

_____

Please tell us about your telephone use

Describe any problems with the work phone _____

How may calls do you handle a day? _____

Do you use a headset? (list brand) _____

What is the model of your work phone?_____

Do you know if it is a digital phone system?_____

Does your phone have volume control?_____

Do you need to answer phones in different areas? _____

Do you have trouble hearing your phone ring?_____

Do you use a cell phone for work? List brand and model #_____

Describe any problems with the cell phone _____

Please tell us about meetings

How many meetings do you attend a month? _____

How many people are in each of those meetings? _____

Are the meetings held in the same or different rooms?_____

Below, sketch the layout of the conference room or table set-up that gives you the most trouble.

Are you attending school or training classes? Please describe

_____

_____

Are you experiencing any problems communicating in class? Please describe

_____

_____

Are you using any support services during classes? Please describe:

_____

_____

Communication Questionnaire

Home Layout

If you have difficulty hearing the phone or doorbell ring at home, please sketch the layout of your home below, indicating where the phone jacks are located. Also list the rooms where you cannot hear the phone or doorbell ring.

First Floor

Second Floor

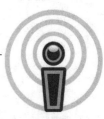

On The Job With Hearing Loss

Please rate the level of difficulty you have in these areas and note details to the right

Use Scale: **A** – Always **O** – Often **S** - Sometimes **N** – Never

Work *Home* *I have difficulty hearing the:*

☐ ☐ Phone ringing - with hearing aid: ☐ in ☐ out ☐ both _____

Working phone jack in the bedroom? ☐ Yes ☐ No _____

☐ ☐ Conversations on the phone - with hearing aid ☐ in ☐ out ☐ both _____

☐ ☐ Alarm clock _____

☐ ☐ Doorbell ringing - with hearing aid:☐ in ☐ out ☐ both _____

☐ ☐ Someone knocking at the door_____

Do you have a working doorbell? ☐ Yes ☐ No _____

☐ ☐ Smoke detector - with hearing aid: ☐ in ☐ out ☐ both _____

☐ ☐ Television/stereo/radio _____

☐ ☐ In one-on-one conversations at banks, work, home, doctors, etc. _____

☐ ☐ In small groups (5 or less) at restaurants, family gatherings, etc. _____

☐ ☐ In large groups (6 or more)_____

☐ ☐ At work with my co-workers _____

☐ ☐ While in a vehicle _____

Please describe the situations that are most difficult for you that you would like to see improved. If you have difficulty at work, be sure to describe those areas also.

Feel free to make any notes and write any thoughts.

1. _____

_____

_____

_____

2. _____

_____

_____

_____

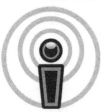

Communication Questionnaire

3. _____

_____

_____

_____

4. _____

_____

_____

_____

5. _____

_____

_____

_____

Is there anything else you would like to tell us about the stress you encounter from your hearing loss or from any other areas that concern you?

_____

_____

_____

_____

_____

_____

_____

_____

Beyond Hearing Aids, Inc.
P.O. Box 353, Florence, KY 41022-0353
1-800-838-1649 v/tty 859-371-1363 Fax
www.BeyondHearingAids.com

Quantity Discounts

For multiple copies of On the Job with Hearing Loss: Hidden Challenges. Successful Solutions, see the discount schedule below. Simply multiply the discount price times the quantity you are ordering. Add 5% of your total order for shipping.

Quantity	List Price	Discount
1 book	$29.95	----
2-14	$25.45	15% off list price
15 +	$22.46	25% off list price

Order From Our Website www.AboutBeckyMorris.com

Call 1-800-838-1649

Formal Communication Assessment Service

It is often desirable to obtain a written formal assessment and report from a qualified third party for case documentation or for additional assistance with a challenging situation.

If you want more information about requesting a formal evaluation and report from Becky Morris or would like to schedule a telephone consultation, please call 1-800-838-1649 to request instructions and the service fee schedule.

Schedule a workshop

Becky Morris is an international workshop presenter who can take technical information and share it in an easy-to-understand and practical format. She has presented at national, regional and state conferences in both the rehabilitation field and hearing health care field.

If you are interested in scheduling training for your staff or workshop for your conference, please call 1-800-838-1649 to request the training/workshop packet.

You can also visit the website www.AboutBeckyMorris.com to review a current bibliography and speaking schedule history.

BONUS !!

You have the tools to identify the challenges in your path. If you would like to spend some time with Becky Morris discussing your personal job challenges and starting a plan to help yourself, be sure and register your book purchase.

Take advantage of this special offer for a personal phone consultation with Becky to explore potential solutions to your specific job challenges. This Special Bonus is valued at $29 and available when you purchase this book.

Register Today for a free 15 minute phone consultation by mailing the coupon below or go to www.onthejobwithhearingloss.com/register

---

Yes Becky! Please contact me to set a 15 minute phone consultation appointment to discuss potential solutions to my personal job challenges related to hearing loss.

Name: _____

Address: _____

_____

Email: _____

Daytime Telephone: _____

Mail this coupon to:
Beyond Hearing Aids, Inc.
P.O. Box 353
Florence, KY 41022-0353

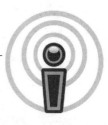
